'*Like many top salon groups, Mahogany believes that education is the way forward and its Mission Statement is to offer all its clients the very best in cut and colour that's available.*'

– Hairdressers Journal

'*A winning combination of commercial elements and futuristic looks.*'

– Estetica UK

'*Mahogany have an uncanny ability to tap into the next big thing in fashion ahead of anyone else. If you are at all interested in modern hairdressing you must follow Mahogany's work.*'

– American Salon, USA

'*Mahogany has become a force to be reckoned with in contemporary hairdressing. The name Mahogany has become synonymous with high standards and quality.*'

– Head, UK

'*Mahogany are extremely innovative and creative; particularly where training is concerned. No international show, exhibition or seminar is complete it seems, without Mahogany putting in an appearance somewhere.*'

– Salon Business, UK

'*Sublime, sensual, smooth! That seems something difficult to achieve, but when you know how easily Mahogany succeed in it day by day you can just ask yourself why you didn't think about it before.*'

– C & C Magazine, Spain

'*Mahogany, the true believers in hairdressing education bring their expertise to all sectors of the industry through publications such as this.*'

– Irish Hairdresser magazine

'*A truly unique cutting technique and a specially innovative use of colour combine for the basis of Mahogany's unmistakable style.*'

– Estetica magazine

'*Cut and colour techniques that are strong and bold for stage presentation but are equally effective when toned down for the salon.*'

– Hairdressers Journal International

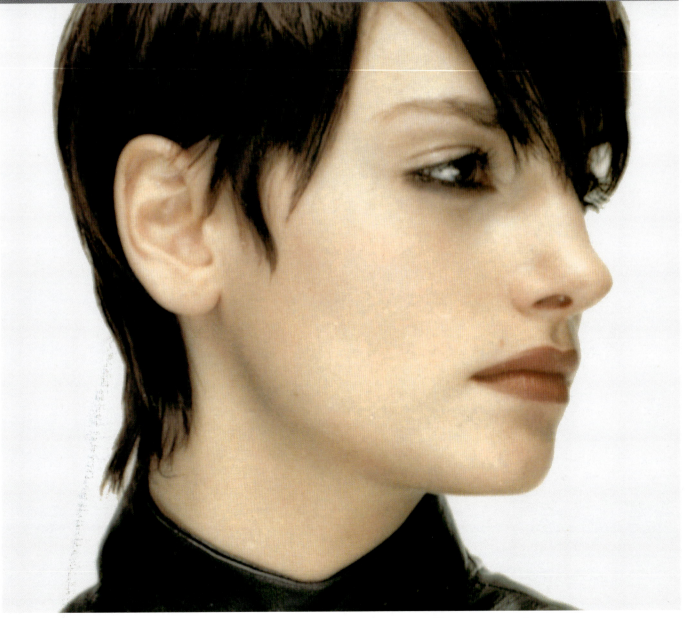

# MAHOGANY
## HAIRDRESSING
## ADVANCED LOOKS

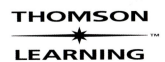

**THOMSON** ™
**LEARNING**

**WELLA**

MAHOGANY

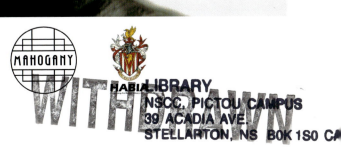

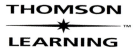

**Mahogany Hairdressing – Advanced Looks**

**Copyright © Richard Thompson and Martin Gannon 2002**

*British Library Cataloguing-in-Publication Data*
A catalogue record for this book is available from the British Library

**ISBN 1-86152-788-8**

**First published 2002 by Thomson Learning**

Designed and typeset by Martin Bristow, London

Printed by in Italy by Canale & C

# Contents

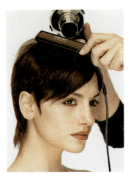
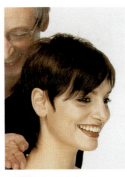
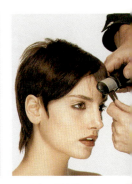

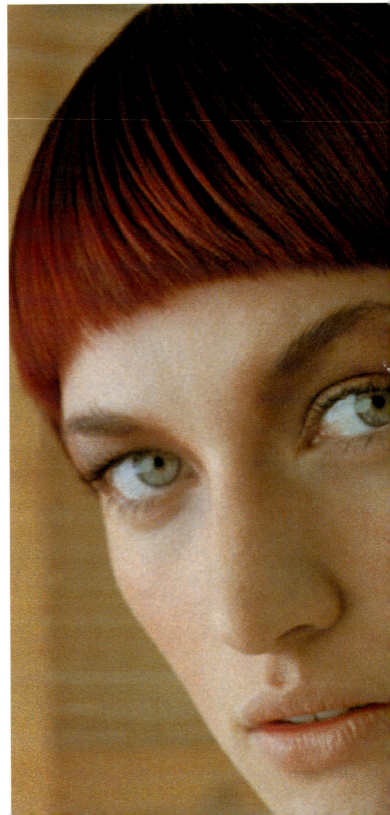

# Step-by-Steps

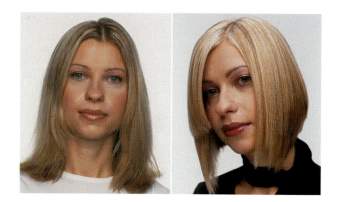

**Deep Division Bob** 8

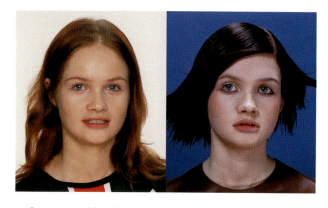

**Channelled Bob** 19

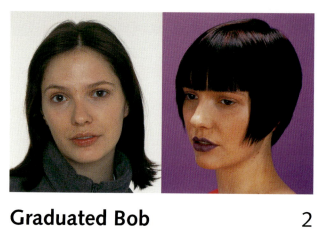

**Graduated Bob** 2

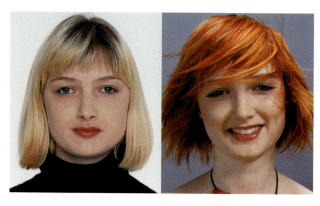

**Swish Bob** 14

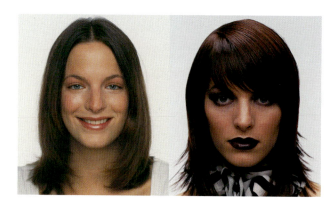

**Freefall Layers** 28

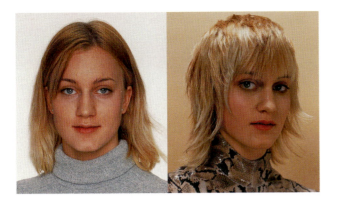

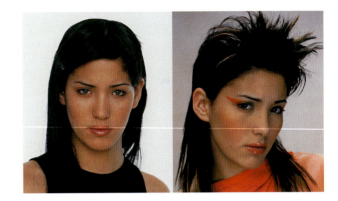

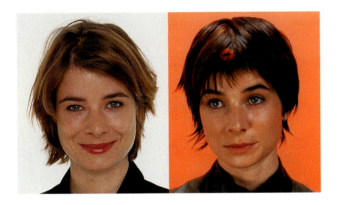

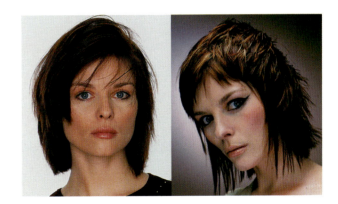

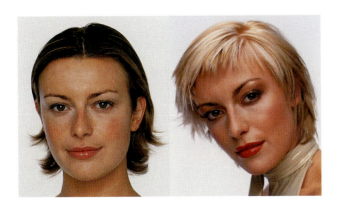

# Step-by-Steps

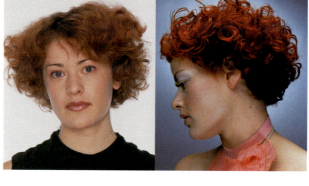

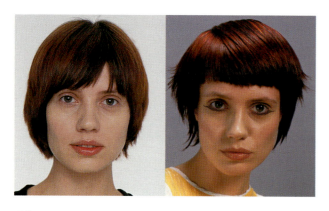

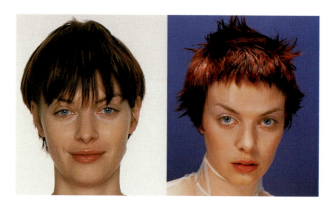

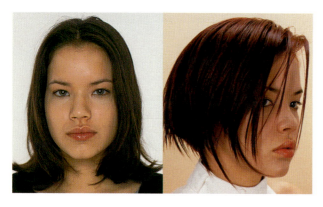

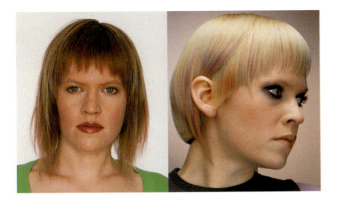

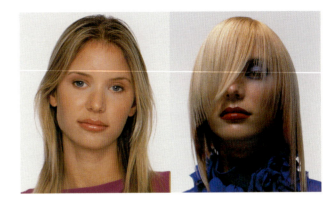

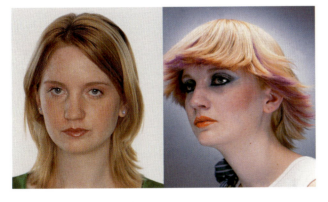

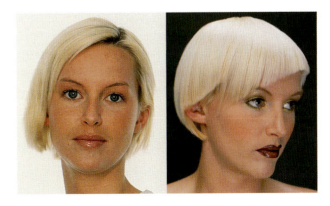

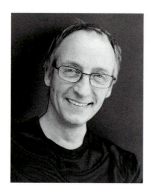

### RICHARD THOMPSON
*Co-Founder and International Creative Director*

Under Richard's Creative Direction, Mahogany has become an internationally respected source of cutting edge British hairdressing. Winner of the AIPP International Avant-Garde Hairdresser Trophy 2000, Richard and the Artistic Team reached the finals of the British Hairdressing Awards 2000. His work includes numerous front covers and makeovers for international trade and consumer magazines and a busy schedule of shows and seminars around the world.

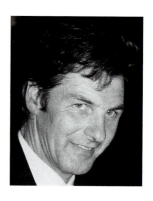

### MARTIN GANNON
*Co-Founder and Marketing/PR Director*

With an experienced background as a hairdresser, Martin has successfully transferred his skills and knowledge to marketing and PR as he directs Mahogany in the development of its profile in the national and international arena. He plays an integral part in developing and breaking new ground for the Mahogany company, always with a keen eye to the future.

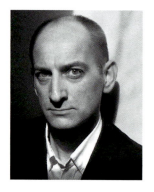

### RUSSELL BARKER
*Commercial Director*

Russell has played an integral role in the commercial success of Mahogany since its inception. After ten year as part of the creative directorship of Mahogany, Russell began to concentrate on the commercial aspects of the business. He is primarily responsible for managing over a hundred Mahogany staff, the export of Mahogany's trade products and the general financial management of the company.

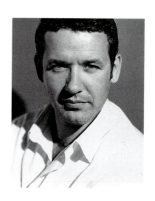

### COLIN GREANEY
*UK Creative Director*

Colin began his training at Mahogany in 1981 and quickly forged a reputation for creative innovation. Heading Mahagany's flagship salon in London, Colin is one of the distinguished winners of the British Hairdressing Awards. His position with Mahogany has taken him all over the world presenting shows and seminars to large hairdressing audiences and he regularly contributes to trade and consumer magazines. More recently, he has evolved as a popular television personality and has a loyal celebrity clientele.

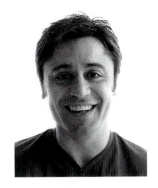

### ANTONY LICATA
*Salons Creative Director*

Antony started his training with Mahogany in 1984 and is now responsible for the training direction of all Mahogany salons. Mahogany's acclaimed training programme won the British Training Award in 1999 and Antony's directorship in the four salons and the new Mahogany Training Academy ensures a clear artistic direction is adhered to throughout the company. Antony regularly presents Mahogany's work at shows and seminars internationally.

### MARK CREED
*Director of technical Development*

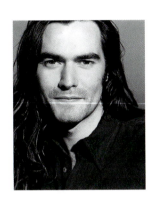

Finalist in the prestigious British Hairdressing Awards as Best British Colour technician 2000, Mark is a highly acclaimed expert in the fields of colour and perm, travelling internationally to demonstrate his skills. Since starting his career with Mahogany in 1984 his consistent development of unique and commercial techniques has become the creative rock base for Mahogany's colour and perm training system and development of their professional products.

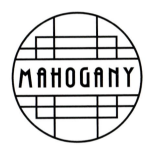

## Salons at:

17 St George Street
Hanover Square
London W1S 1FJ
Telephone 020 76293121

5 Turl Street
Oxford OX1 3DQ
Telephone 01865 248143

30 Little Clarendon Street
Oxford OX1 2HU
Telephone 01865 552494

5 Market Street
Oxford OX1 3EF
Telephone 01865 790245

Academy Education
Telephone 01865 791332

Central Office:
5 Turl Street
Oxford OX1 3DQ
Telephone 01865 791332
Fax 01865 722454

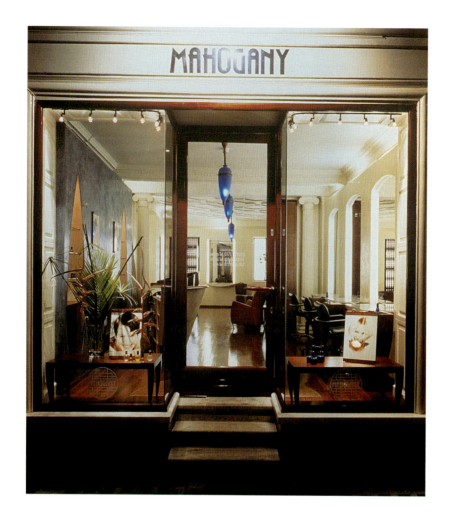

The Mahogany team wish to thank Paul Burley for photography
and Julia Clancey for clothes styling in the Step-by-Steps.

# Preface

Hardly a day goes by when the press aren't talking about the latest haircut on this or that celebrity or model. Hairdressing has become such a high profile industry to work within that we, as hairdressers, owe it to our clients to constantly educate ourselves in the latest techniques in order to offer them the very best of modern hairdressing.

It has been three years since our first book *Steps to Cutting, Colouring and Finishing Hair* presented Mahogany's interpretation of the classic looks of our time and it remains as important as ever to master these basics, but where do we go from there? *Advanced Looks* previews the cut and colour techniques that the Mahogany team use every day to keep our clients coming back and spreading the word.

Taken to their extreme, these looks grace the catwalks at our international shows and seminars, but the same looks are diluted for everyday use in our four busy salons and are vital to our business. Our location – in the heart of London opposite the *Vogue* offices and a stone's throw from the Bond Street designer boutiques – keeps us constantly on our toes and our clients demand the very best.

London is a constant source of inspiration with its rich cultural and aesthetic diversity and Mahogany's work within the music and fashion industries provides us with not only ideas, but also clients and a promotional tool. Entertainers like Radiohead, Bryan Adams and Billie Piper, models such as Erin O'Connor and actors like Greta Scacchi and Nick Moran are regular clients and reinforce Mahogany's position as an inspirational salon group through their own celebrity status in magazines and on TV. The power of the press can never be overestimated and as such Mahogany has its own press office dedicated to keeping our name in the public eye.

Mahogany's close relationship with Wella is of great importance. We have worked together for many years producing professional products and creating images for editorial and advertising purposes. Their constant support has undoubtedly contributed to our success as winners of the AIPP International Avant Garde Hairdresser of the Year Trophy 2000 and the British Training Award 1999.

The Mahogany team hope you enjoy *Advanced Looks* and if there is just one idea you take and commercialise for your own business then we feel as though our project has been worthwhile. Enjoy!

The Mahogany team

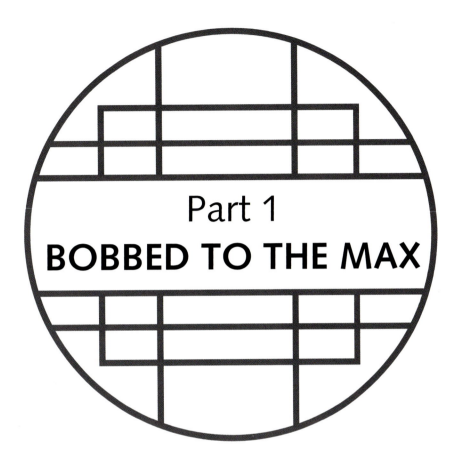

# Part 1
# BOBBED TO THE MAX

*The bob shape is a timeless classic.*
*We create the nouveau classic*

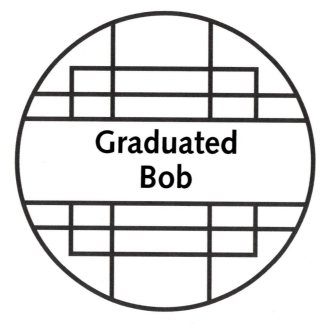

**Graduated
Bob**

*Graduated outline
complemented by a square-cut fringe*

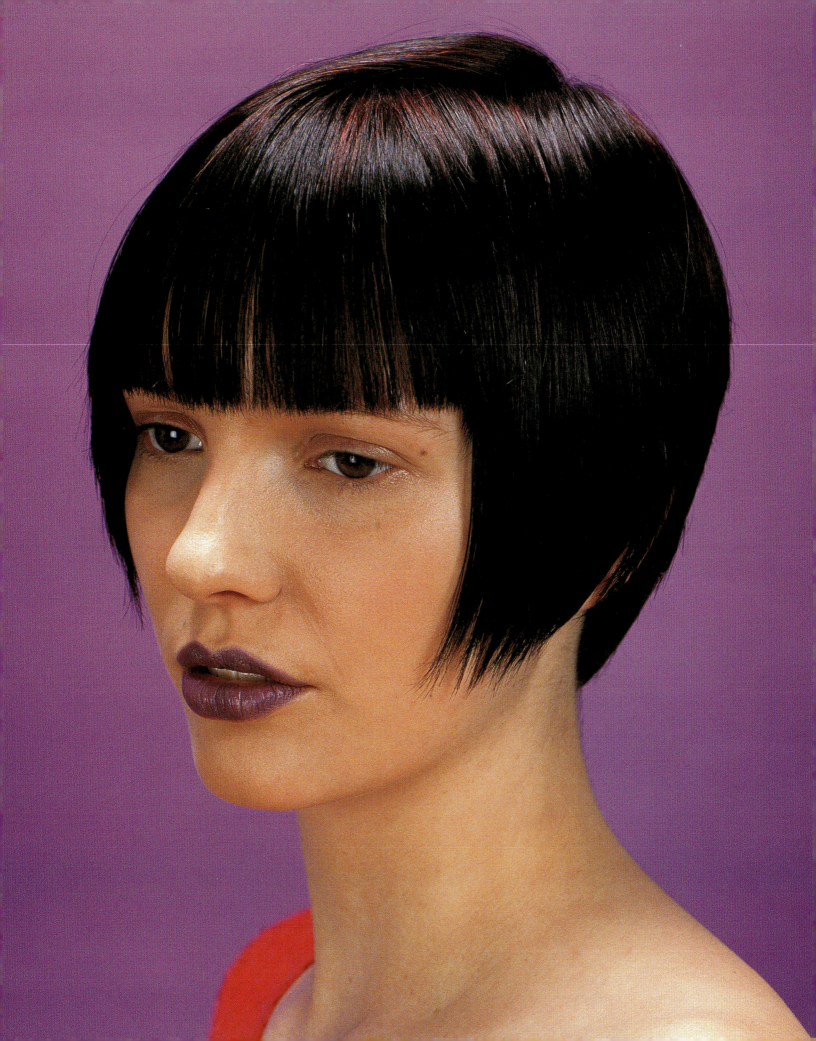

# Cutting

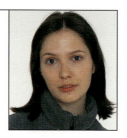

*Our model's hair is a one-length, grown-out, straight bob. After consultation, it was decided to go for a short, graduated shape with a fringe and the colour would be dark and rich to emphasise the shape.*

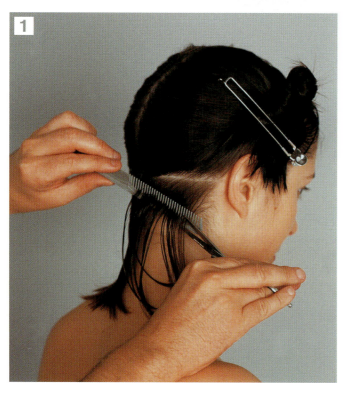

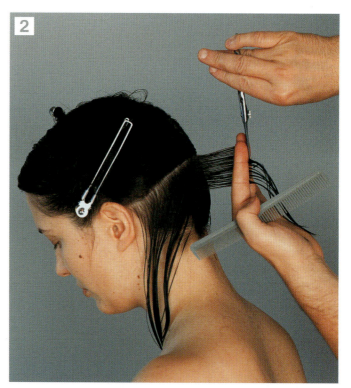

**1** Section out first panel and scissor over comb into the neck.

**2** Taking the second panel, start a new line and graduate a length that will cover the hairline.

**3** Move into the side panel, continuing the line you started at the back.

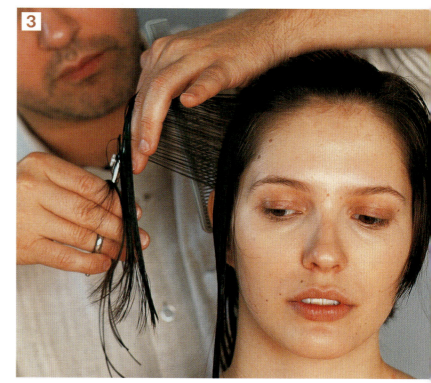

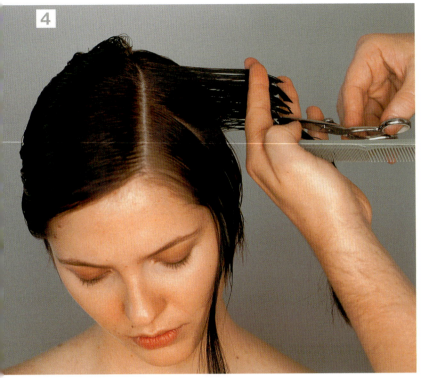

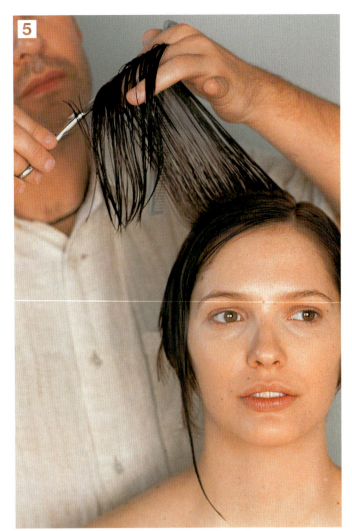

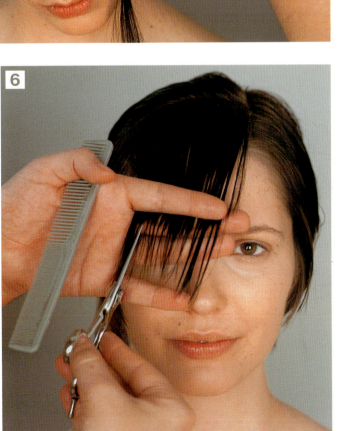

**4** When the side panels are complete point ends for a broken outline.

**5** Connect in the top panels.

**6** Cut a square fringe to length of the eyebrow.

The hair is now ready for colouring.

5

# Colouring

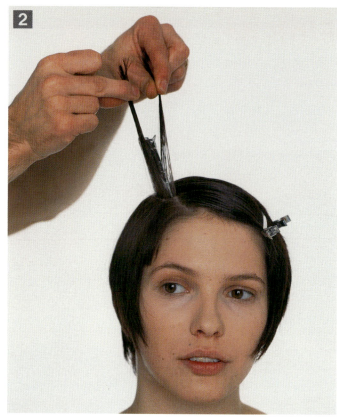

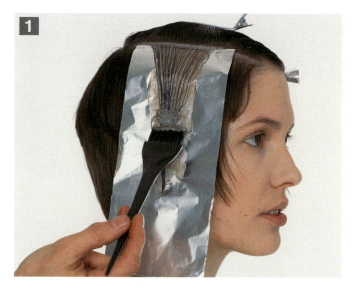

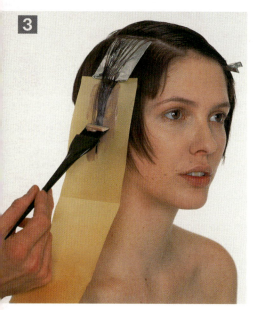

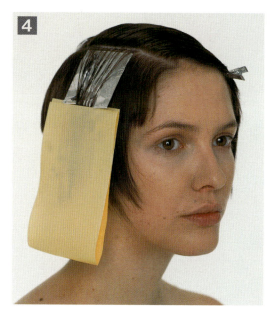

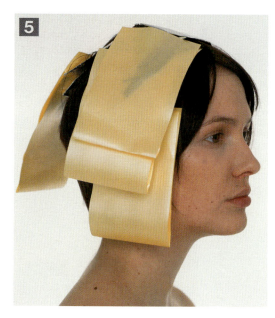

**1** A fine section of hair is taken from the parting and tinfoil is placed underneath. Hair is coloured using Wella Koleston Perfect 55/55 Intense Mahogany mixed with 6% Wella Welloxon Perfect Creme Developer from roots to ends.

**2** Tinfoil is then folded in the usual way to form a neat packet. Two fine sections from front and behind are taken.

**3** The two fine sections are then combined and placed on top of a Colour Wrap and coloured using Wella Koleston Perfect 44/65 Intense Damson Red mixed with 9% Wella Welloxon Perfect Creme Developer.

**4** The Colour Wrap is then folded to seal.

**5** Continue working through the top layers using the same technique. Allow the colour to process, then shampoo and condition as usual.

# Finished Look

The hair is dried and finished using Wella SP Styling Spray Lotion with a small amount of Wella SP Mould & Shine Creme.

## Products used

Wella Koleston Perfect:
    55/55 Intense Mahogany
    44/65 Intense Damson Red

6% Wella Welloxon
Perfect Creme Developer

9% Wella Welloxon
Perfect Creme Developer

Wella SP Styling Spray Lotion

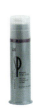

Wella SP Mould & Shine Creme

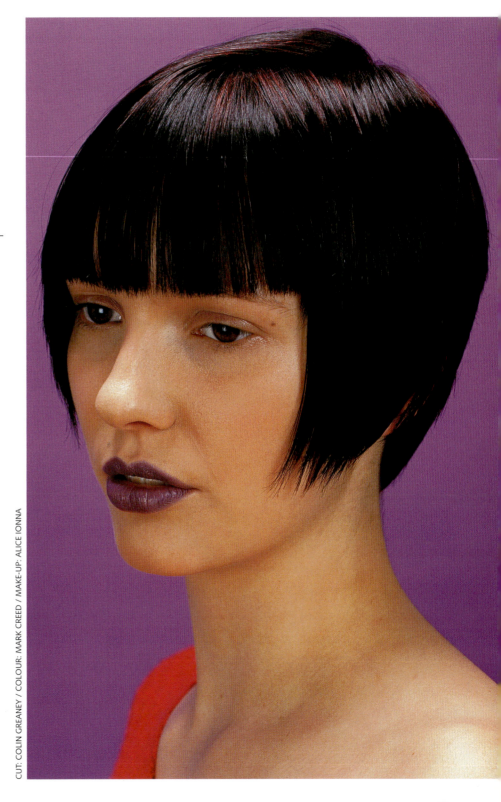

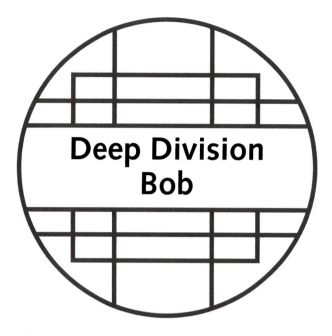

**Deep Division
Bob**

*Graduated outline enhanced by deep divisional
panels that are cut freehand*

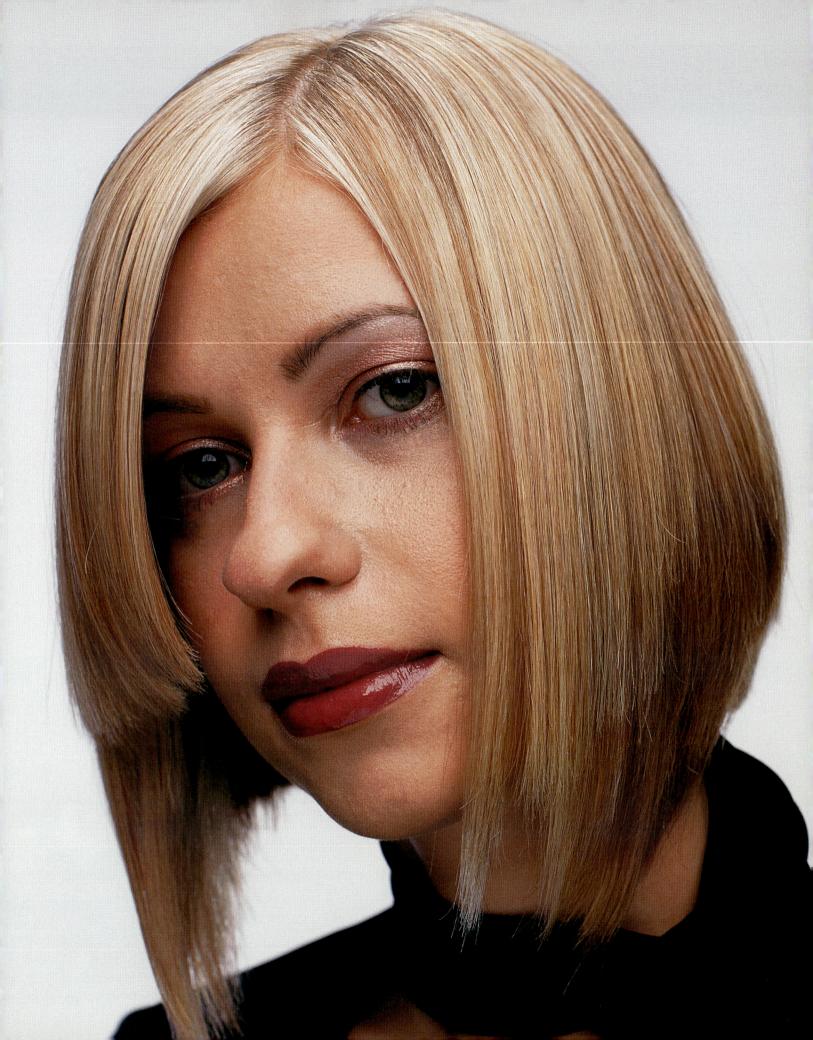

# Cutting

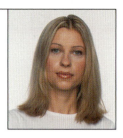

*Our model has one-length, shoulder-length hair with very light blonde highlights. She wants a more interesting version of a classic bob in lighter blonde without having a full head of colour.*

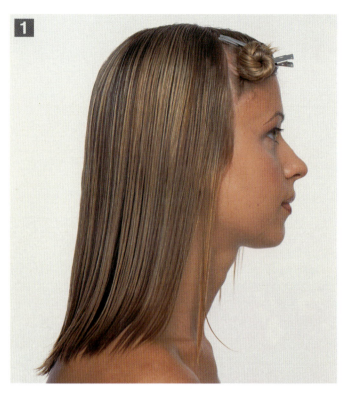

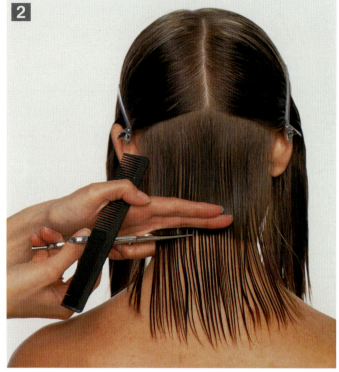

**1** A triangular panel is sectioned off at the front.

**2** Establish the outline length.

**3** Work up to the crown using a horizontal graduation technique. This creates a gentle bevel to the outline.

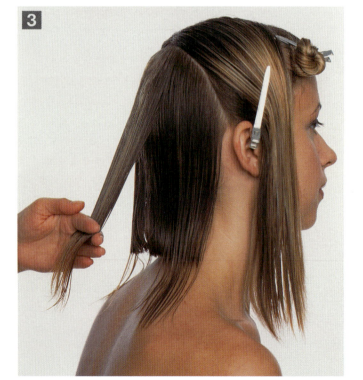

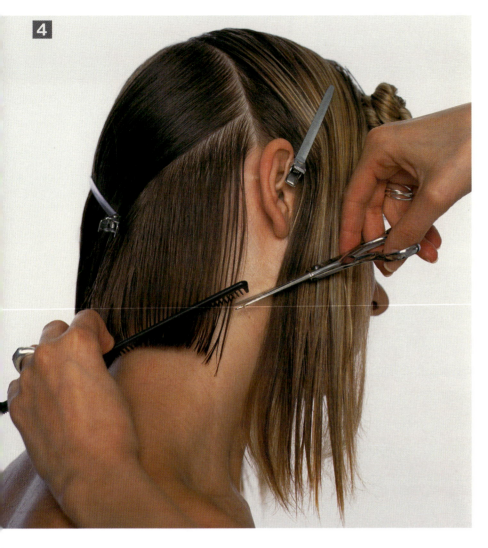

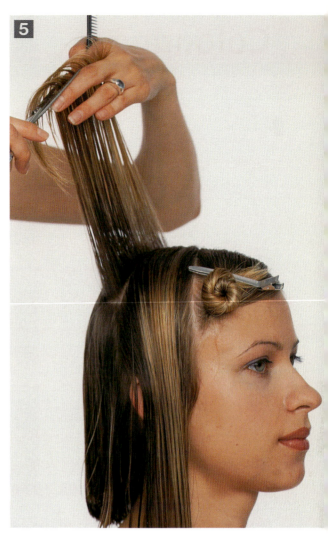

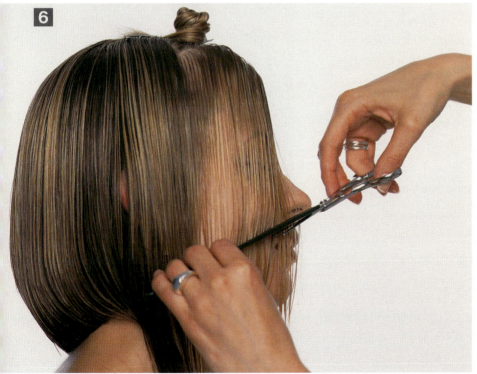

**4** Cut off the back corner, aiming the angle to come in line with the cheekbones.

**5** Layer off the top corner using the top length of the horizontal graduation as your guide.

**6** Let down the first section of the front triangular panel. Cut a line to meet the back line from the cheekbone. Dry the hair and then visually tailor the last remaining panel according to personal taste.

# Colouring

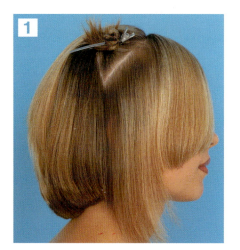

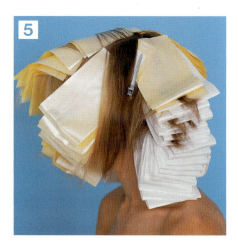

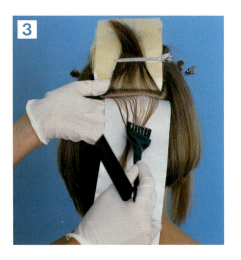

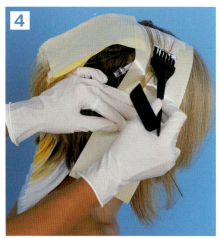

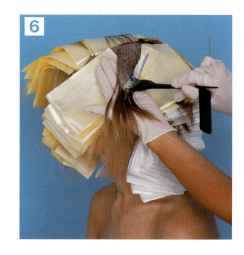

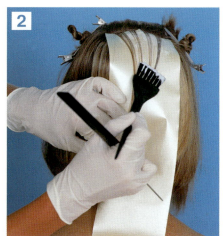

**1** Section out a triangular section, this will be coloured using a different combination of colours.

**2** Taking the first weaved section on the crown use Colour Wraps and apply Wella Koleston Perfect 12/16 Special Soft Ash mixed with 12% Wella Welloxon Perfect Creme Developer. Work down to the occipital bone using this colour.

**3** Weave the under sections from the occipital bone down using Creative Colour Wraps to apply Wella Koleston Perfect 12/17 Special Soft Velvet and Wella Koleston Perfect 9/03 Very Light Beige Blonde mixed in equal parts with 12% Wella Welloxon Perfect Creme Developer.

**4** Work through the whole head using the same technique leaving out the original triangular section.

**5** Triangular section previously left out is now ready to be coloured.

**6** Triangular section is placed on to a Colour Wrap and coloured using Wella Koleston Perfect 12/17 Special Soft Velvet mixed in equal parts with Wella Koleston Perfect 9/03 Very Light Beige Blonde with 12% Wella Welloxon Perfect Creme Developer. This section is sealed with a Colour Wrap to protect the remaining hair.

**7** Allow the colour to process, then shampoo and condition as normal.

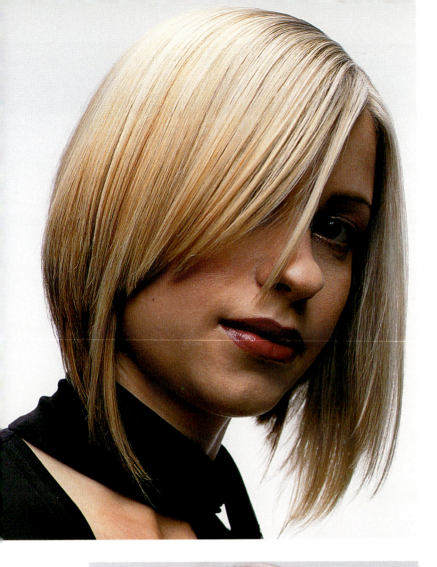

# Finished Look

The hair was dried and finished using a small amount of Wella SP Ends Express.

## Products used

 Wella Koleston Perfect:
    12/16 Special Soft Ash
    12/17 Special Soft Velvet
    9/03 Very Light Beige Blonde

 12% Wella Welloxon
Perfect Creme Developer

 9% Wella Welloxon
Perfect Creme Developer

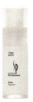 Wella SP Ends Express

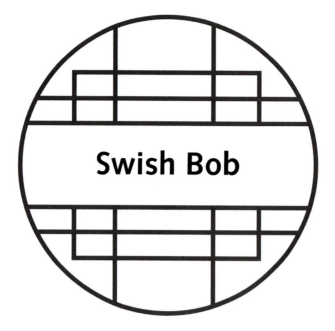

**Swish Bob**

*Extreme layers on the inside to longer outline layers create this in-out swish bob*

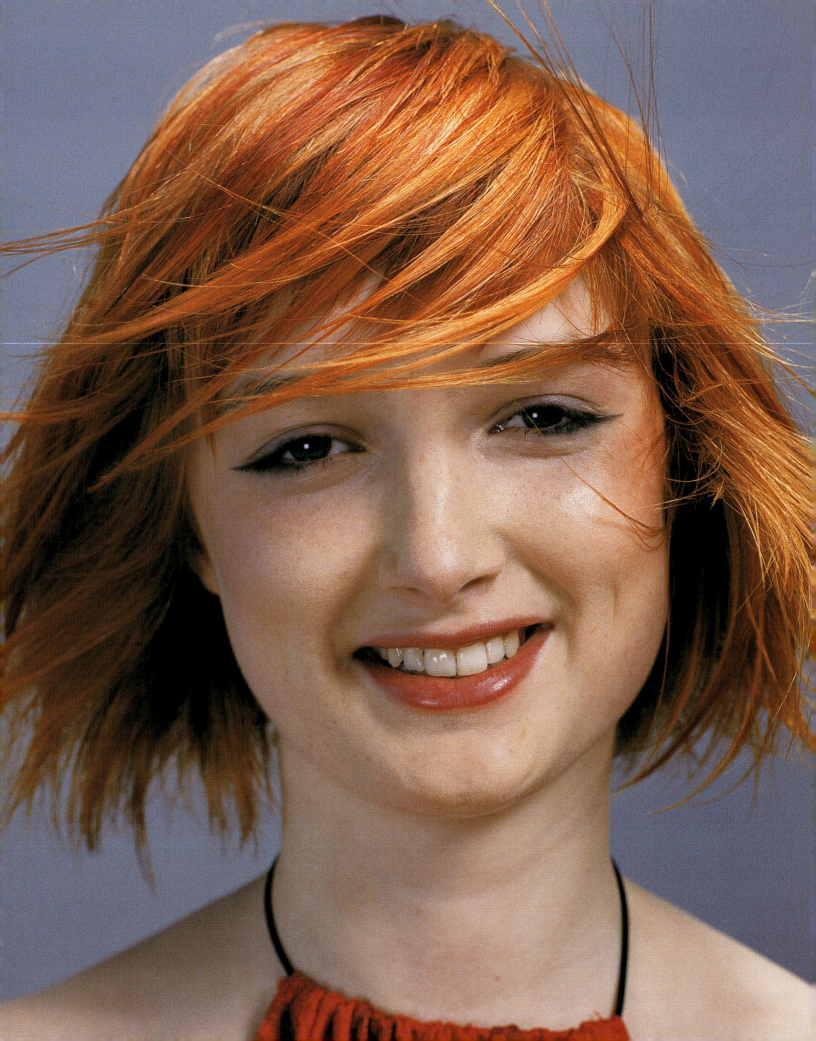

# Colouring

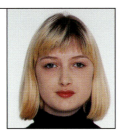

Our model's hair was a classic square bob with a full fringe. She wanted a total change of cut and colour. After consultation, she decided on a very layered wispy shape, coloured with a bright rich copper. The model had coloured her hair at home using a high lift tint blonde colour. She now has a regrowth of approximately 5 cm. Her natural colour is a 7/0 Medium Blonde.

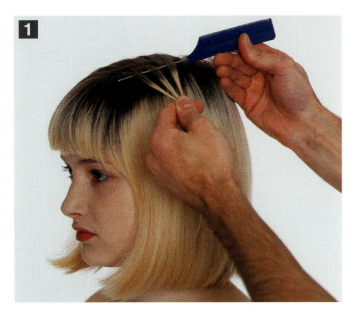

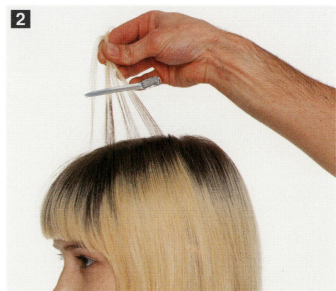

**1** + **2** A section was woven from the parting and clipped out of the way. This section will be used later.

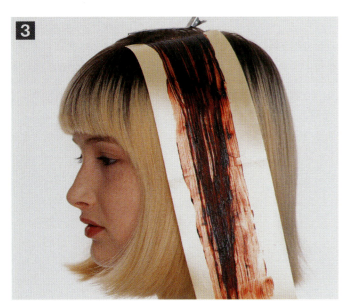

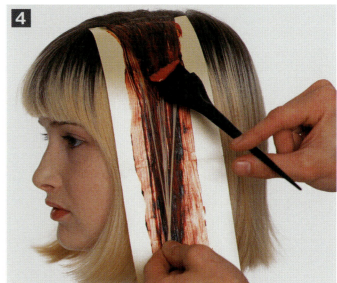

**3** + **4** Take a fine slice of hair underneath the previous section, place on a Colour Wrap and apply Wella Koleston Perfect 55/55 Intense Mahogany mixed with 6% Wella Welloxon Perfect Creme Developer, from roots to ends.

The first woven section is then unclipped and placed directly on top of the first section and coloured using Wella Koleston Perfect 88/43 Vibrant Celtic Copper mixed with 6% Wella Welloxon Creme Developer. These colours are allowed to fuse together.

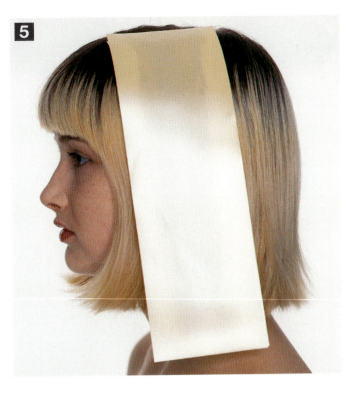

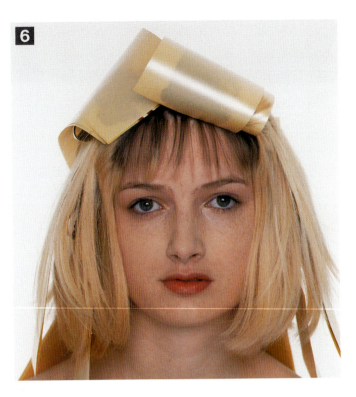

**5** + **6** A Colour Wrap is placed on top of section, to seal. Repeat this technique working throughout the top layers.

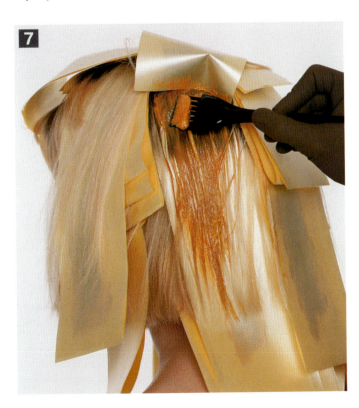

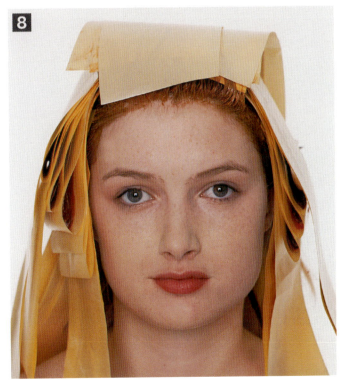

**7** + **8** Apply Wella Koleston Perfect 77/43 Intense Celtic Copper mixed with 6% Wella Welloxon Perfect Creme Developer throughout the rest of the hair.

Allow the colour to process, then shampoo and condition as normal.

# Cutting

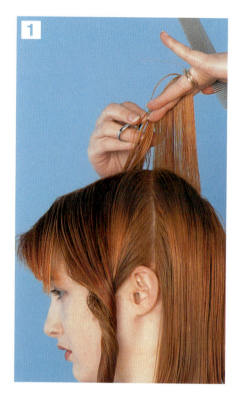

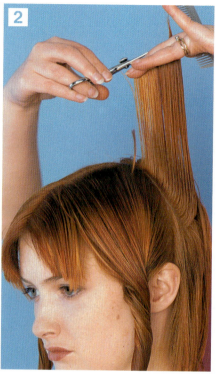

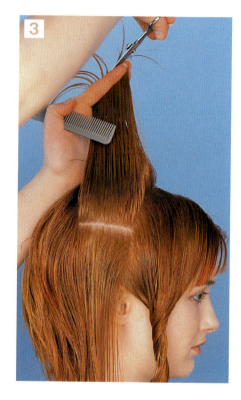

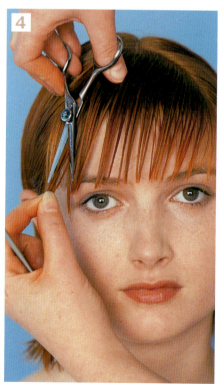

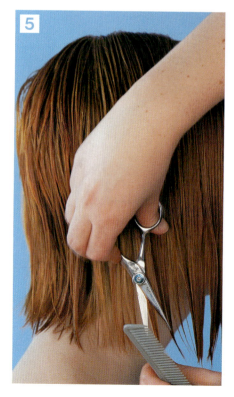

**1** Section hair from crown to top of ear. Taking your first section decide on the crown length and angle towards the outline.

**2** Continue working through the back, in segments, to just behind the ear.

**3** Using your first section as your guide angle outwards to meet the outline.

**4** Establish the length of fringe and slide cut for texture.
Note: The top lengths do not check in with the fringe length.

**5** Slide cut into the outline until the desired separation of texture is achieved.

# Finished Look

Wella Koleston Perfect:
55/55 Intense Mahogany
88/43 Vibrant Celtic Copper
77/43 Intense Celtic Copper

The hair was dried using Styling Spray Lotion and finished with Wella SP Mould & Shine Creme.

6% Wella Welloxon
Perfect Creme Developer

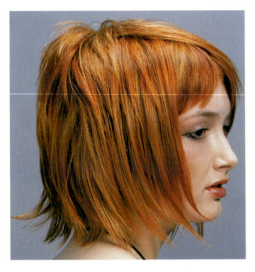

Wella SP Styling Spray Lotion

Wella SP Mould & Shine Creme

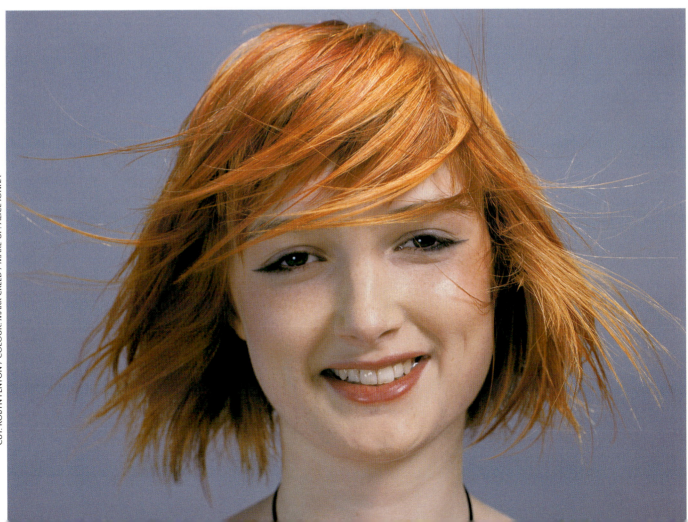

CUT: ROBYN FENTON / COLOUR: MARK CREED / MAKE-UP: ALICE IONNA

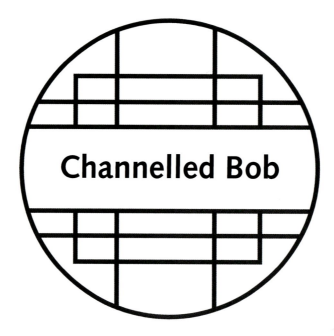

**Channelled Bob**

*Using a subtle channelling technique,
maximum freedom of movement is created*

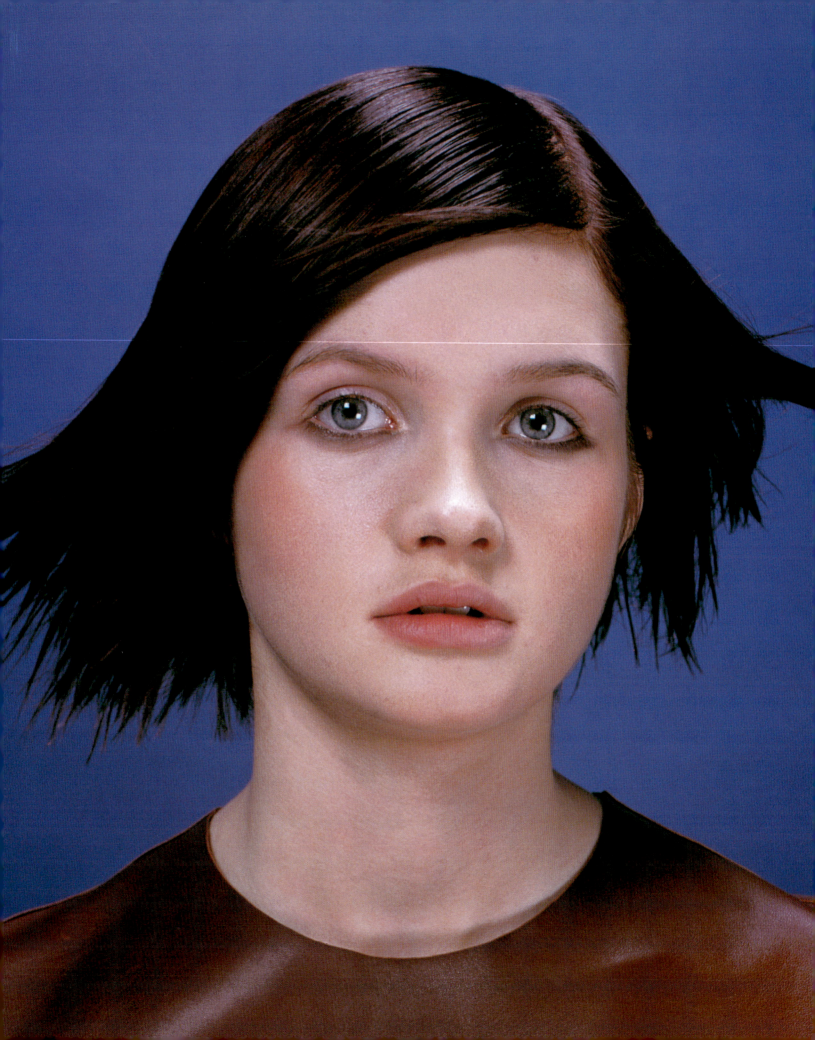

# Colouring

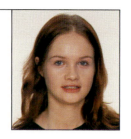

*Our model's hair was shoulder length and from the jaw line down was quite damaged. After consultation, it was decided to go for a shattered bob effect and to take the colour to a rich nutty dark brown. The model's hair is 7/10 medium blonde, which has a 3 cm regrowth from an old home-done tint. Hair texture is fine.*

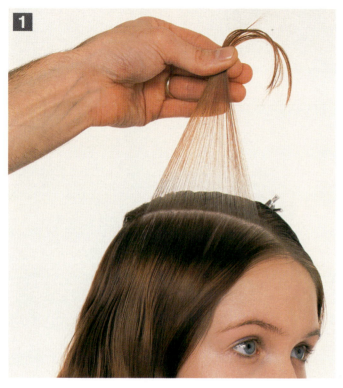

**1** A fine mesh of hair is taken from an offset parting. Note this section is wider than a normal section.

**2** + **3** A Creative Colour Wrap is placed underneath the section and Wella Koleston Perfect 6/75 Rich Heather mixed with 6% Wella Welloxon Perfect Creme Developer is applied from roots to ends.

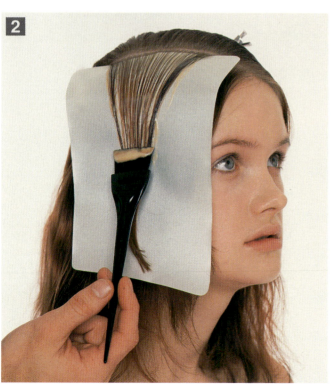

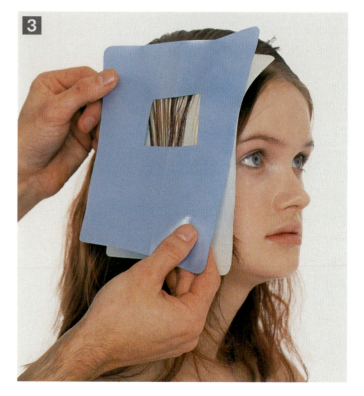

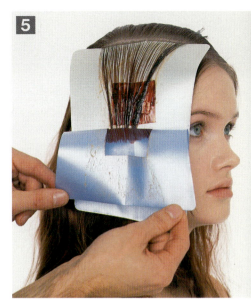

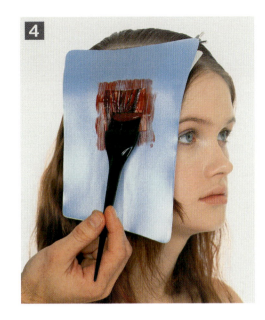

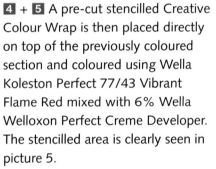

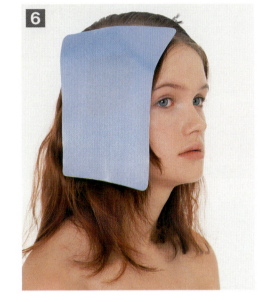

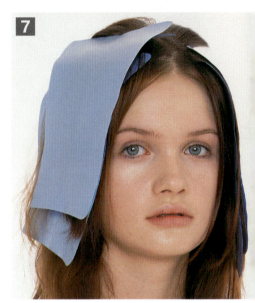

**4** + **5** A pre-cut stencilled Creative Colour Wrap is then placed directly on top of the previously coloured section and coloured using Wella Koleston Perfect 77/43 Vibrant Flame Red mixed with 6% Wella Welloxon Perfect Creme Developer. The stencilled area is clearly seen in picture 5.

**6** A Creative Colour Wrap is placed on top of the stencilled Colour Wrap to seal.

**7** Repeat this technique through the top sections with the Colour Wraps approximately 1 cm apart.

**8** + **9** Wella Koleston Perfect 6/7 Rich Velvet Blonde mixed with 6% Wella Welloxon Perfect Creme Developer is applied to the rest of the hair and then left to process. When finished, shampoo and condition as normal.

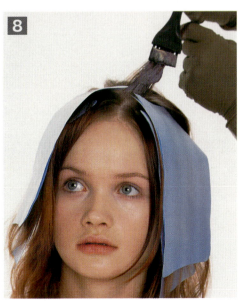

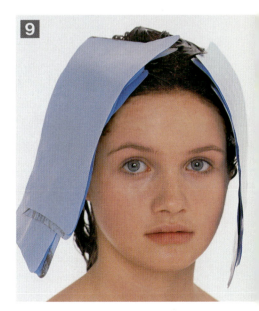

# Cutting

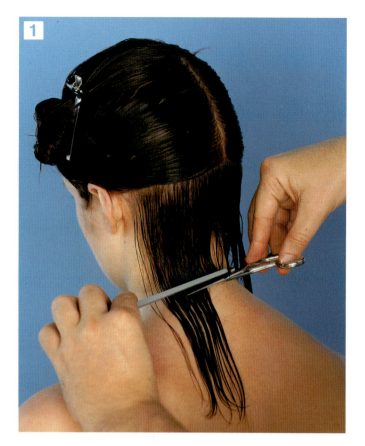

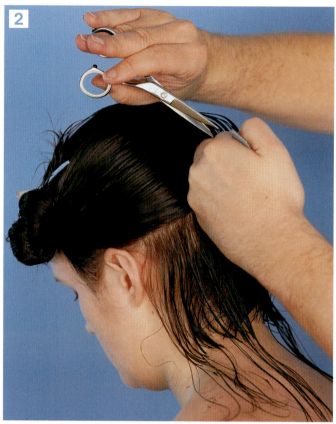

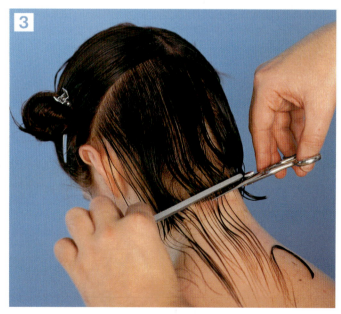

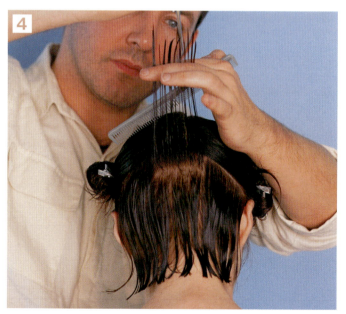

**1** Cut first section to the desired outline length.

**2** Lift up the panel and vertically cut the lengths to the desired point length. This creates your first channel.

**3** Take down the next panel cutting it again to the outline length.

**4** Next section is cut to the length of the first point cut section, again creating a channel.

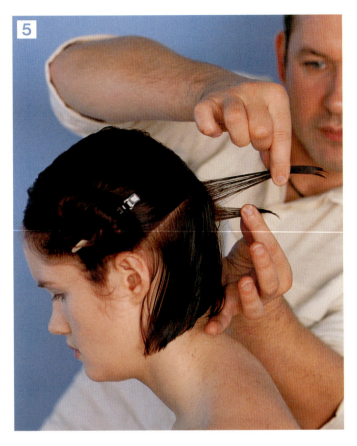

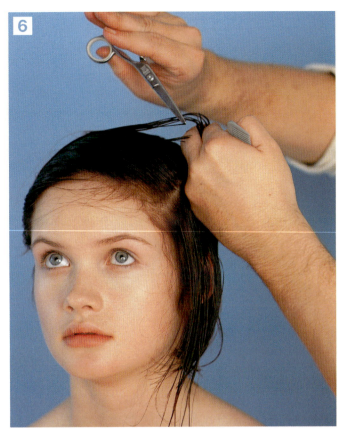

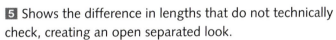

**5** Shows the difference in lengths that do not technically check, creating an open separated look.

**6** Continue into the sides.

**7** Note the difference in lengths.

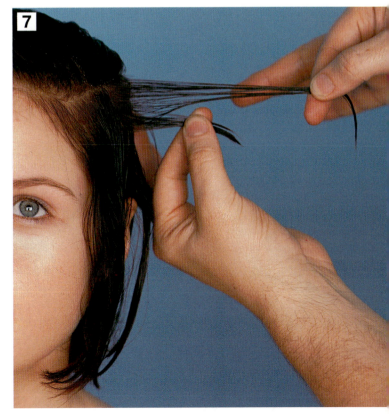

25

# Finished Look

The hair was dried using Wella SP Texturising Mousse and finished using Wella SP Mould & Shine Creme.

Wella Koleston Perfect:
6/75 Rich Heather
77/44 Vibrant Flame Red
6/7 Rich Velvet Blonde

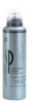

6% Wella Welloxon
Perfect Creme Developer

Wella SP Texturising Mousse

Wella SP Mould & Shine Creme

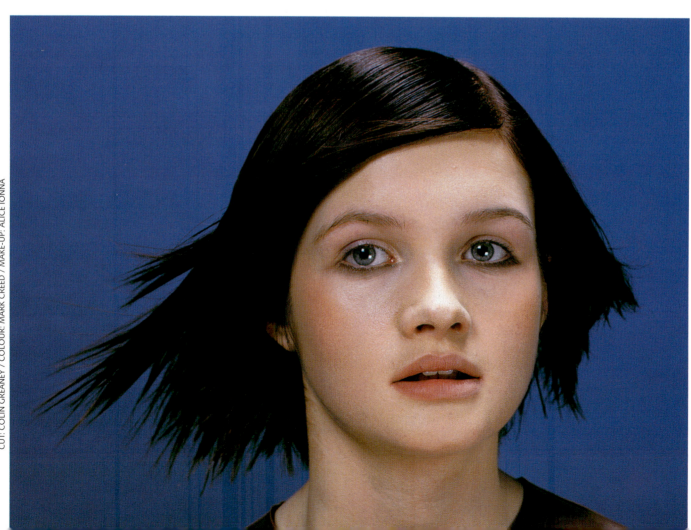

CUT: COLIN GREANEY / COLOUR: MARK CREED / MAKE-UP: ALICE IONNA

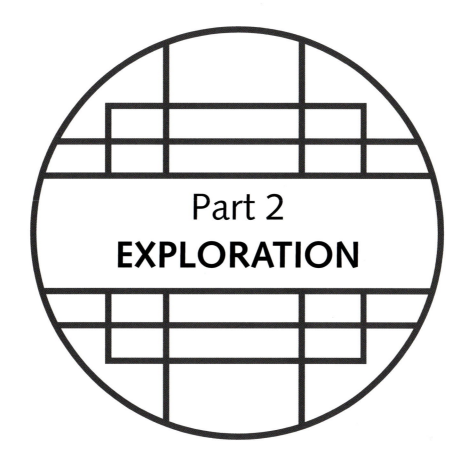

# Part 2
# **EXPLORATION**

*Explore the methods and uses of layering –
classic disconnection and texturising.*

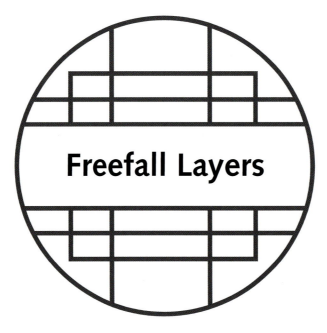

# Freefall Layers

*Layering creates freedom of movement
and the ability to change the look*

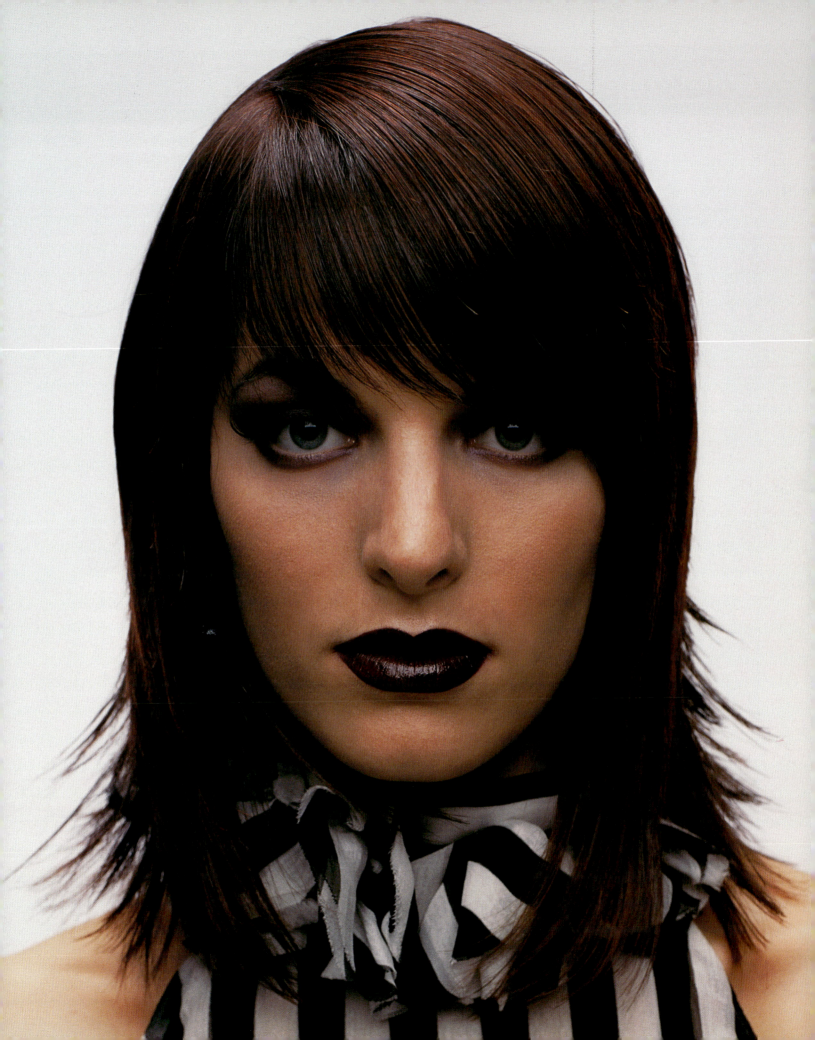

# Colouring

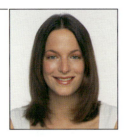

*Our model has shoulder-length hair. She wants to keep the length, but have a more exciting, layered shape. We layered the hair and created an asymmetric front that can be worn to either side.*

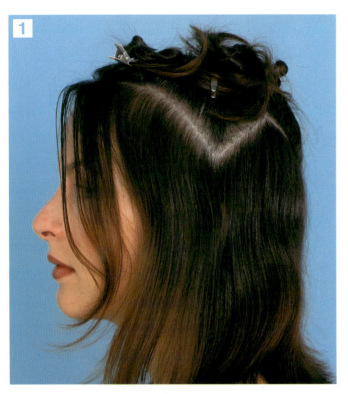

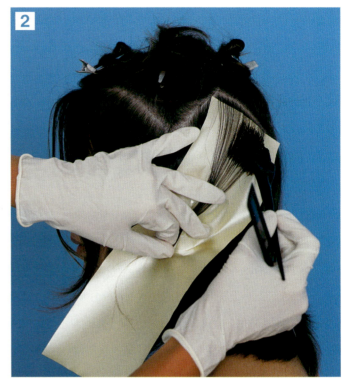

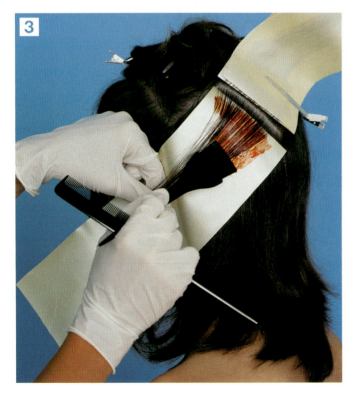

**1** Top hair is separated and sectioned, using a zig-zag pattern, around the head.

**2** + **3** Take a fine slice directly underneath the zig-zag section and place onto a Colour Wrap. Colour from roots to ends using Wella Koleston Perfect 7/75 Warm Heather mixed with 6% Wella Welloxon Creme Developer. Continue working around the head using this slicing technique on the zig-zag section.

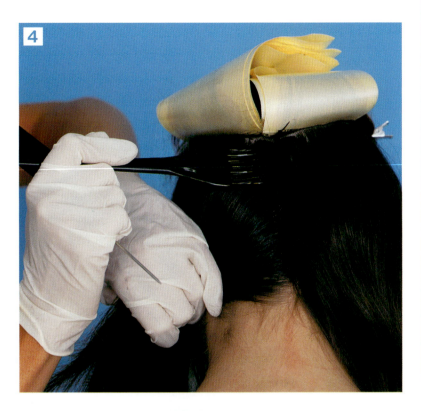

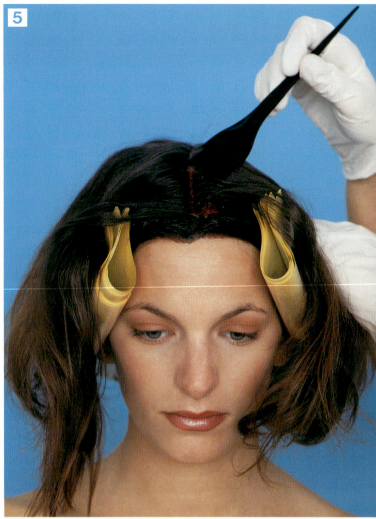

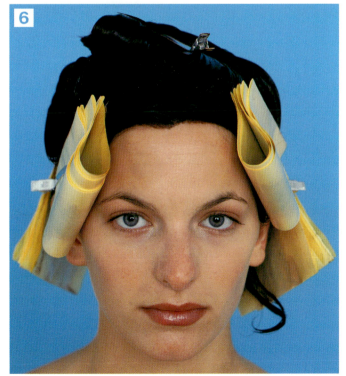

**4** After completing the zig-zag section, colour the underneath sections using Wella Color Touch 3/0 Dark Brown mixed with Wella Colour Touch Intensive Lotion Developer.

**5** Colour the rest of the hair using Wella Color Touch 8/40 Irish Copper mixed with Wella Color Touch Intensive Lotion Developer.

**6** Allow colour to process, then shampoo and condition as normal.

# Cutting

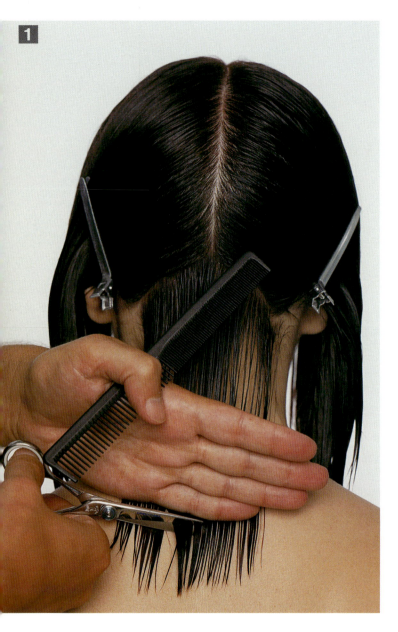

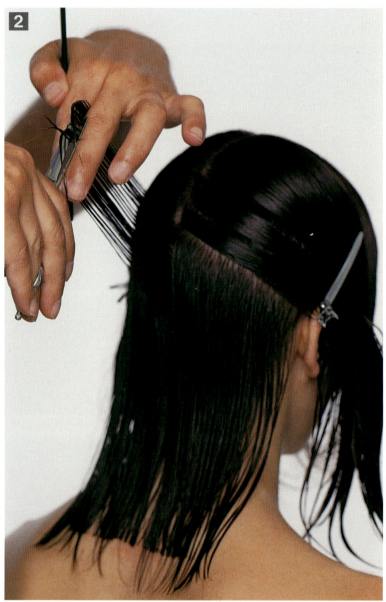

**1** Cut a square outline to the desired length.

**2** Starting at the centre back, layer the hair parallel to the head shape. Continue on both sides cutting each section parallel to the head.

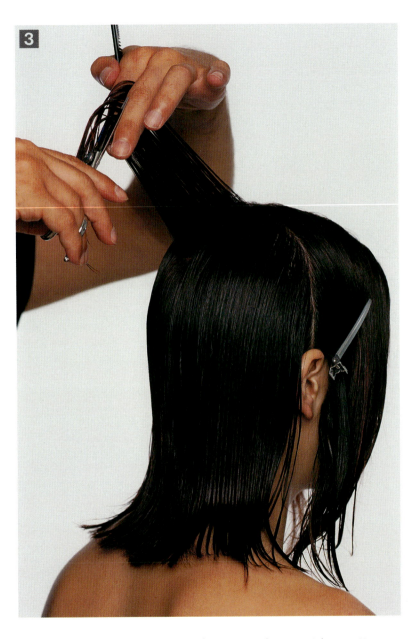

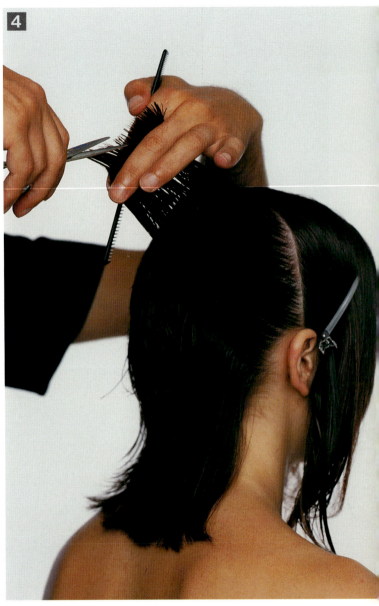

**3** Using your previously cut panel as a guide, continue the line to achieve your length on the crown.

**4** Overdirect the last section to the level of the head shape overstepping the line to leave a corner behind the ear.

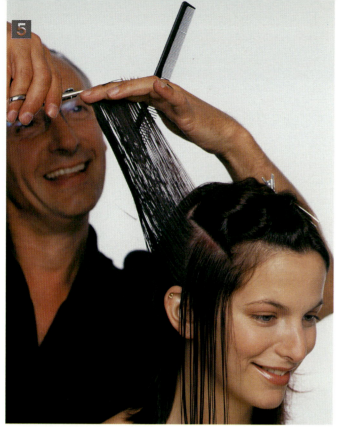

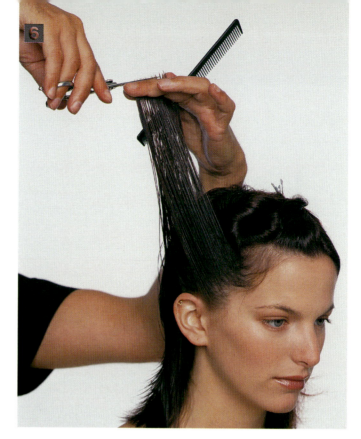

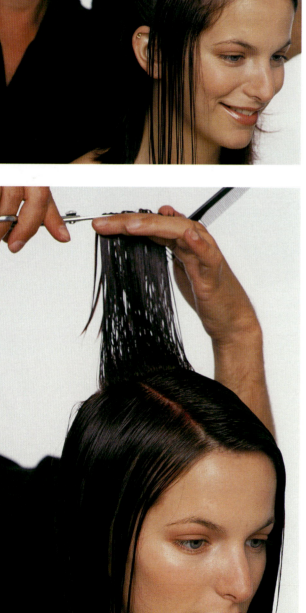

**5** Work into the side panel using the last section of the back panel as your guide.

**6** Overdirect the last section in line with the top of the ear.

**7** Check in the top layers.

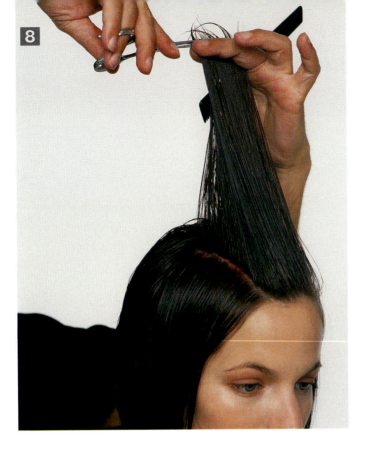

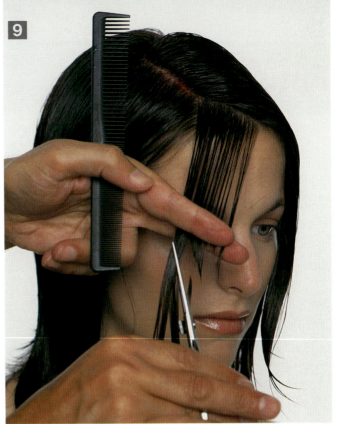

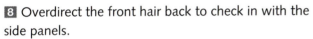

**8** Overdirect the front hair back to check in with the side panels.

**9** Establish the length of the fringe cutting deep V-sections into the ends.

**10** Continue overdirecting the fringe to the left side to build up length on the right, creating an asymmetric result. Continue until the hair runs out.

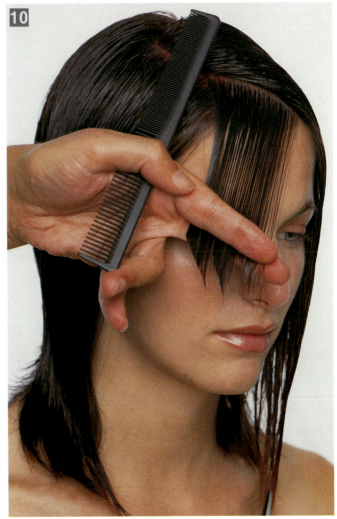

# Finished Look

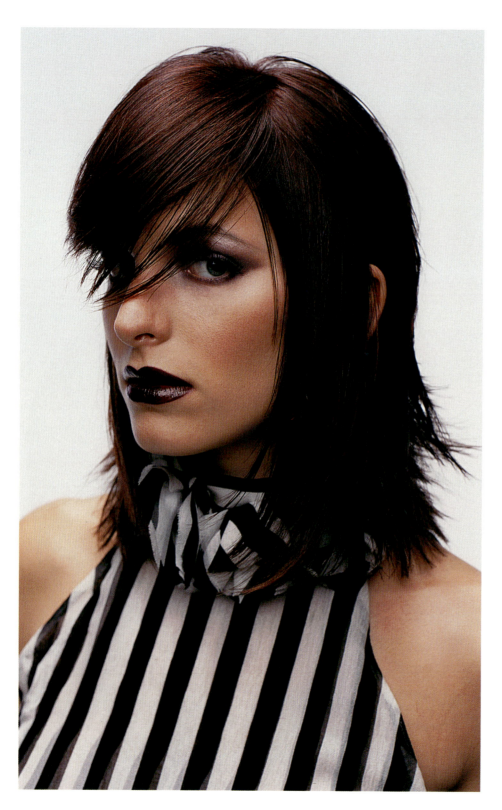

The hair was dried using Wella SP Controlling Spray and dressed with Wella SP Ends Express.

## Products used

Wella Color Touch
3/0 Dark Brown
8/40 Soft Irish Copper

Wella Color Touch
Intensive Lotion Developer

Wella SP Controlling Spray

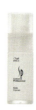

Wella SP Ends Express

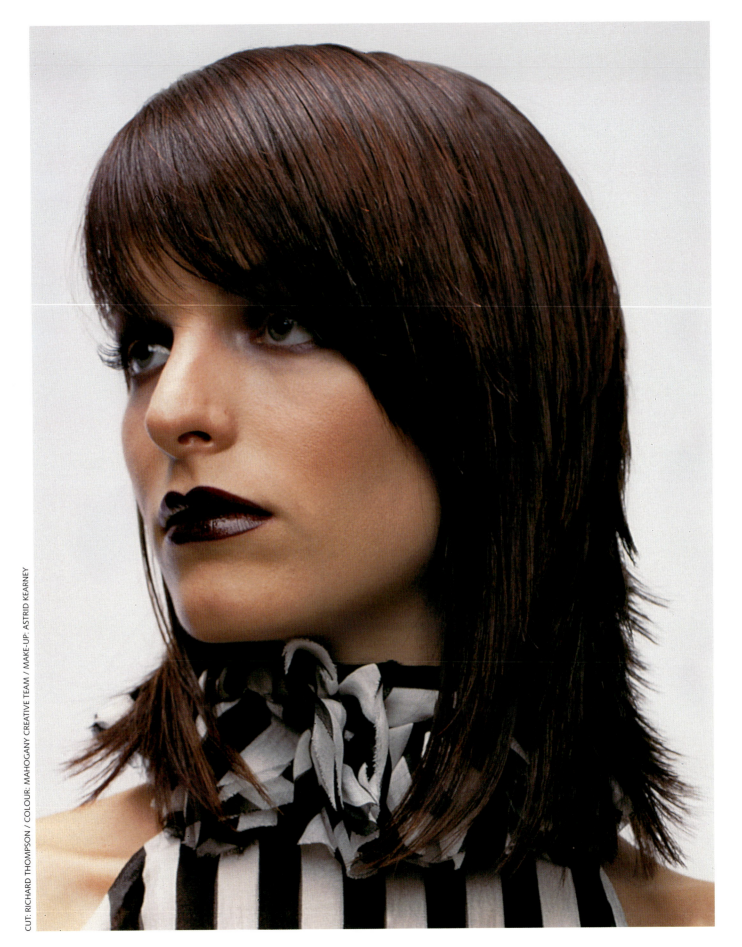

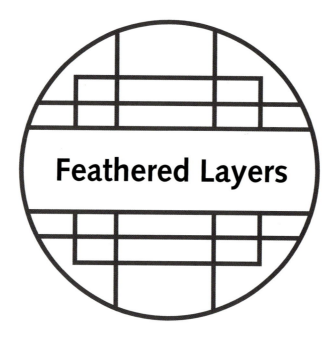

**Feathered Layers**

Steep point cut layering creates a light, feathery outline

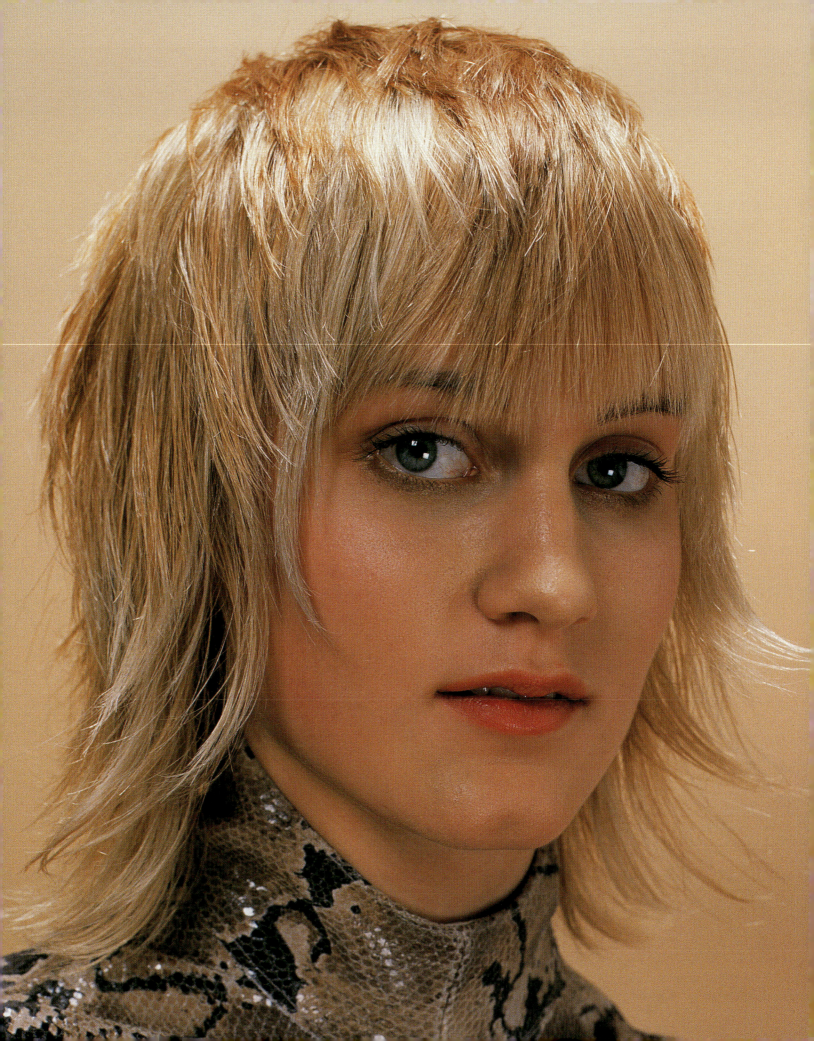

# Cutting

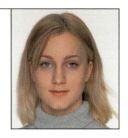

*Our model's hair was shoulder length with a few layers around the face. After consultation, it was decided to stay blonde and have a very layered 'Rock Chic' image.*

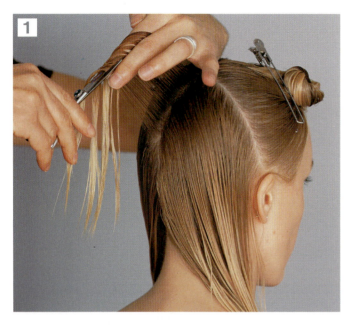

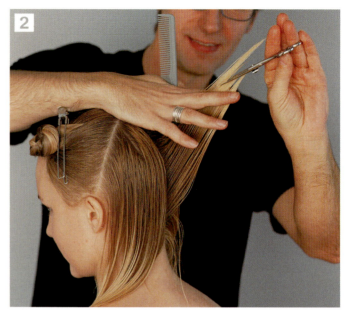

**1** Section the back panel from crown to top of the ear and take your first section parallel to the head shape.

**2** From 2 cm above the occipital bone cut at a very steep angle to create a feathery outline.

**3** The difference in length from the crown to the outline.

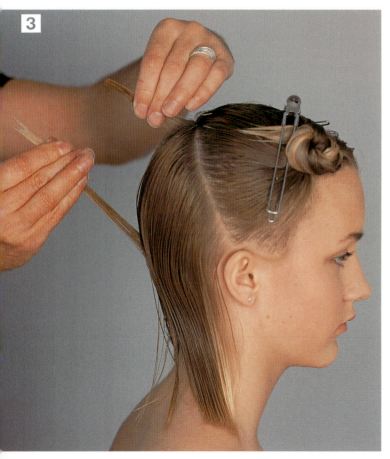

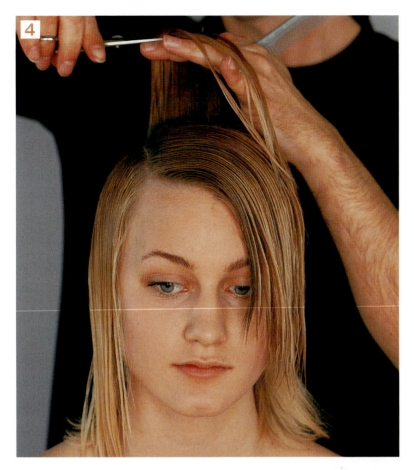

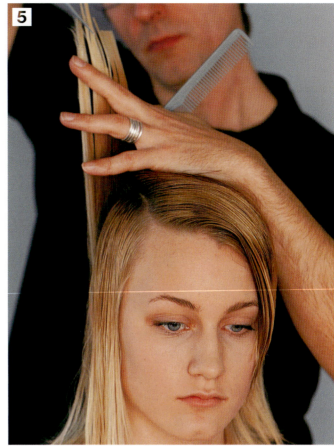

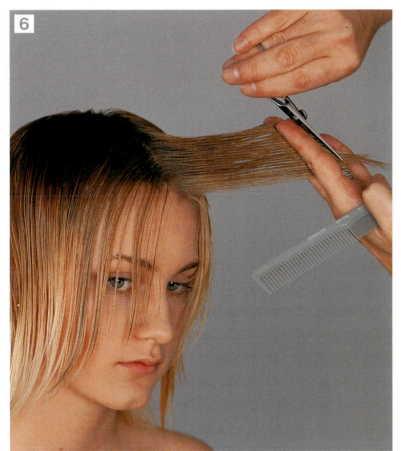

**4** Section out the top panel and cut square using your first section as your guide.

**5** Angle out the lower panel and cut towards the outline.

**6** Angling outwards from the crown create the length of the fringe; this will be checked forward as well, to create a long in-the-eyes fringe.

The hair is now ready for colouring.

# Colouring

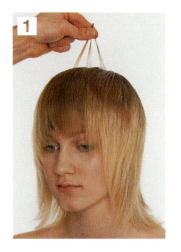 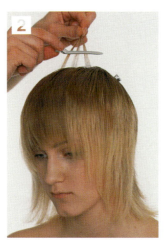 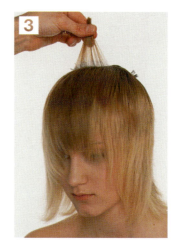 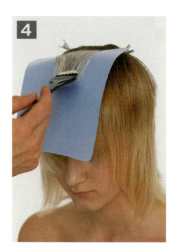

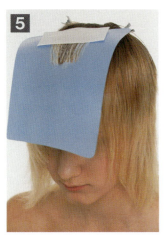 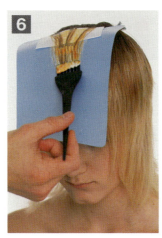 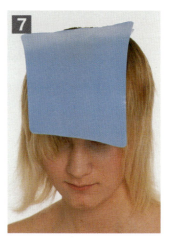 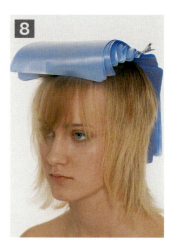

**1** A fine mesh is taken from the crown. Note that this section is woven and slightly wider than a normal section.

**2** The section is then clipped out of the way with a sectioning clip. This section will be used later in this technique.

**3** Another fine mesh is taken directly behind the first section. This section is the same width as before but this time it's a slice as opposed to a weave.

**4** A Colour Wrap is placed underneath the slice of hair and Wella Koleston Perfect 10/0 Lightest Blonde mixed with 6% Wella Welloxon Perfect Creme Developer is applied from roots to ends.

**5** A small piece of Colour Wrap is then placed near the root area. This will act as a barrier, producing a varying brightness of colour on the same section.

**6** The first woven section is released from the sectioning clip and laid directly on top of the Colour Wraps. This section is then painted from roots to ends with Wella Koleston Perfect 9/3 Very Light Golden Blonde mixed with 9% Wella Welloxon Perfect Creme Developer.

**7** A Colour Wrap is placed on top of the section to seal.

**8** This technique is repeated through the top layers. Leave colour to process, then shampoo and condition as normal.

# Finished Look

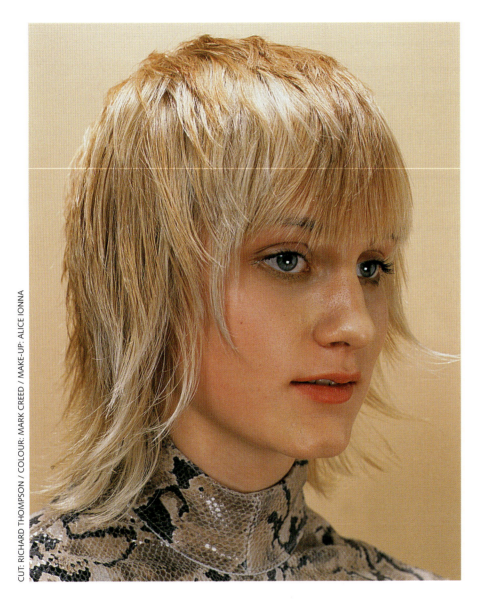

CUT: RICHARD THOMPSON / COLOUR: MARK CREED / MAKE-UP: ALICE IONNA

The hair was dried using Wella SP Styling Spray Lotion and finished using Wella SP Mould & Shine Creme.

## Products used

Wella Koleston Perfect:
   10/0 Lightest Blonde
   9/3 Very Light Golden Blonde

6% Wella Welloxon
Perfect Creme Developer

9% Wella Welloxon
Perfect Creme Developer

Wella SP Styling Spray Lotion

Wella SP Mould & Shine Creme

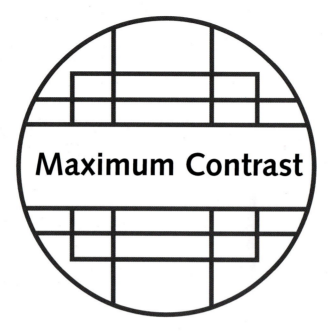

**Maximum Contrast**

*Short and long hair together is always commercial.
This look is a modern interpretation of maximum
contrasting layers*

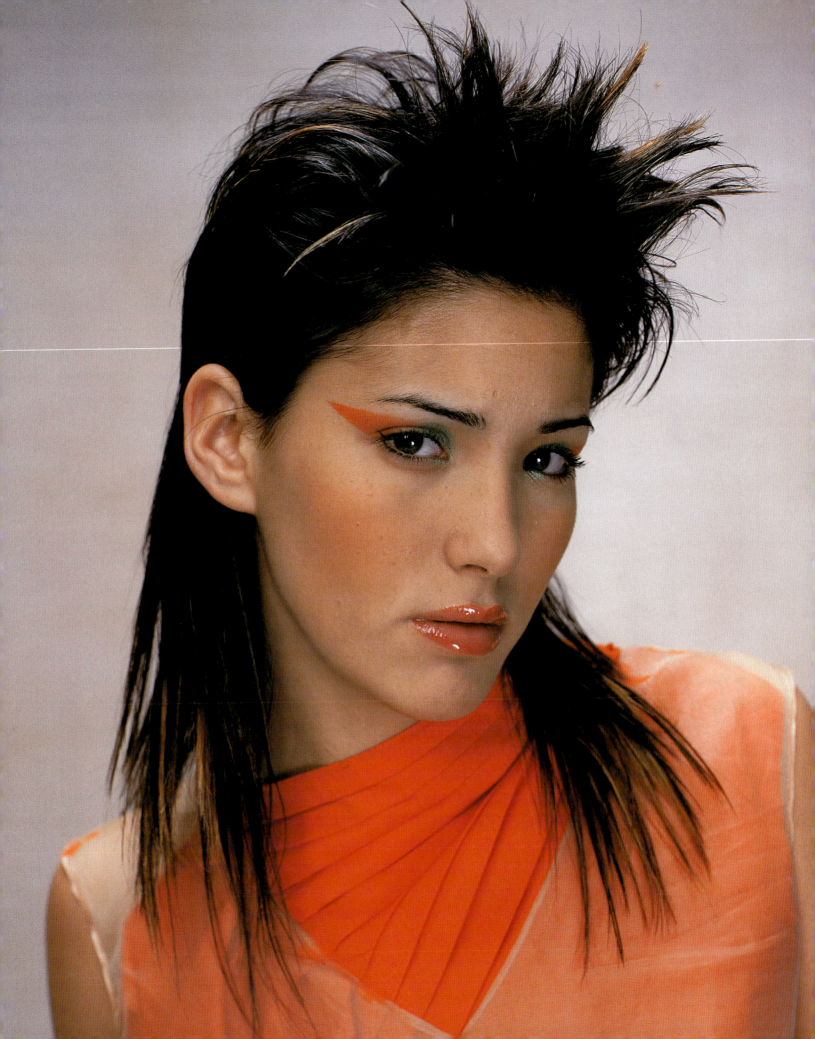

# Colouring

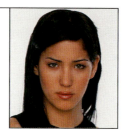

*The model's hair was long with a grown-out fringe. She had done the colour herself and the result was uneven and too dark. She wanted lighter hair and a layered 'Rock Chic' cut.*

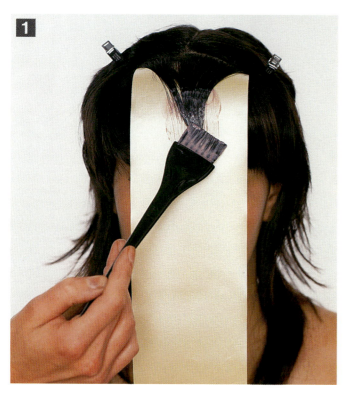

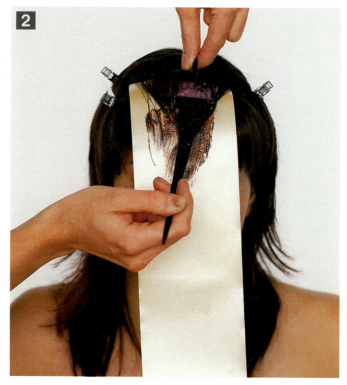

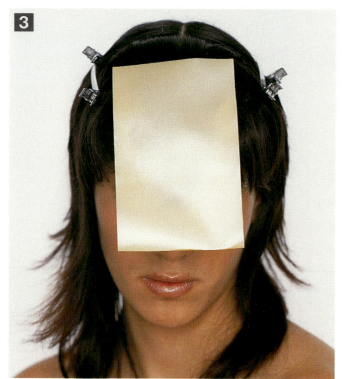

**1** Starting at the fringe, take a section, place on a Colour Wrap and colour mid-lengths to ends.

**2** Take a section 2 cm back from the first section, clipping away the hair in between the section and place on first Colour Wrap. Apply colour to the ends using Wella Koleston Perfect 7/43 Warm Celtic Copper mixed with 6% Wella Welloxon Perfect Creme Developer.

**3** Fold and seal Colour Wrap.

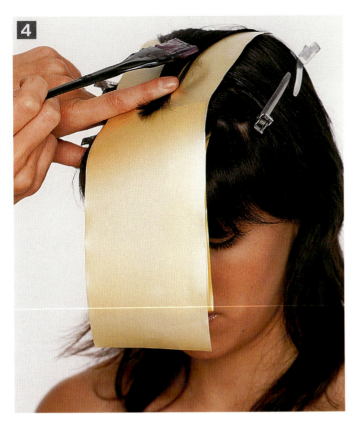

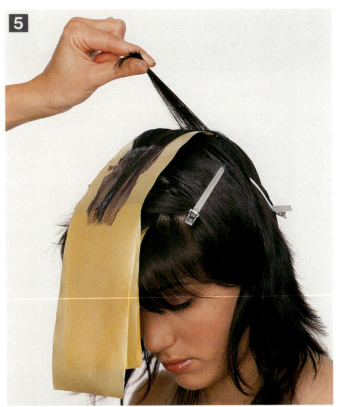

**4** Continue this technique through all the top sections.

**5** The second section is pulled over in between sections and placed on previous sections' Colour Wraps.

**6** Apply colour to ends using Wella Koleston Perfect 10/1 Lightest Ash Blonde mixed with 12% Wella Welloxon Perfect Creme Developer.

**7** Seal and continue through entire head. Allow colour to process, then shampooo and condition as normal.

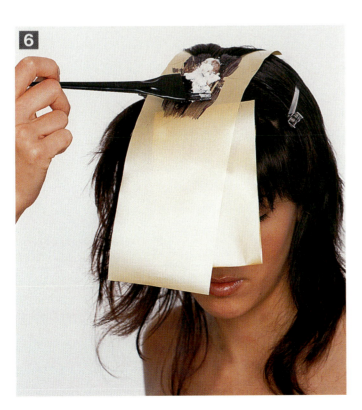

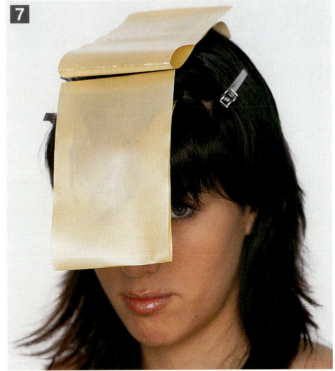

# Cutting

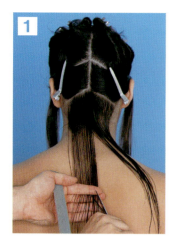

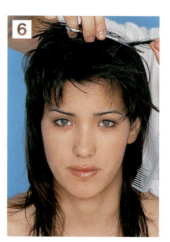

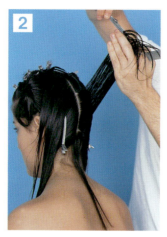

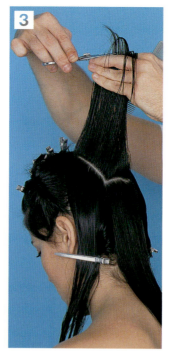

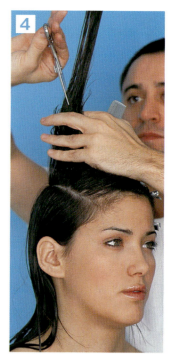

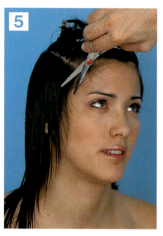

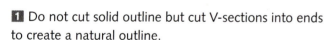

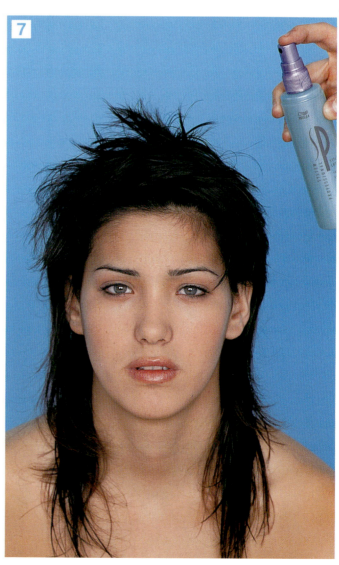

**1** Do not cut solid outline but cut V-sections into ends to create a natural outline.

**2** Layer underneath panel into the outline length.

**3** Continue up to 2 cm below the crown.

**4** Start a new line, angle section steeply from crown to a visual length that will hang over the previously cut length of the preceding section.

**5** Cut front outline close to hairline at temple and slide out to the long back lengths.

**6** Increase the texture on the top sections by twisting and slide cutting the twist, starting approximately 2 cm from the root.

**7** Apply Wella SP Styling Spray Lotion and finger dry.

# Finished Look

Finish with Wella SP Sculpting Gel for the ultimate texture and separation.

## Products used

Wella Koleston Perfect:
7/43 Warm Celtic Copper
10/1 Lightest Ash Blonde

6% Wella Welloxon
Perfect Creme Developer

12% Wella Welloxon
Perfect Creme Developer

Wella SP Styling Spray Lotion

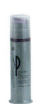

Wella SP Sculpting Gel

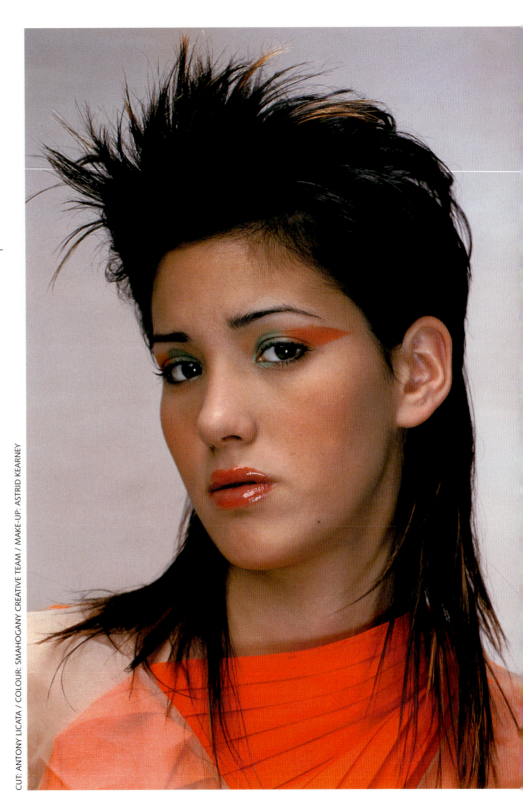

CUT: ANTONY LICATA / COLOUR: SMAHOGANY CREATIVE TEAM / MAKE-UP: ASTRID KEARNEY

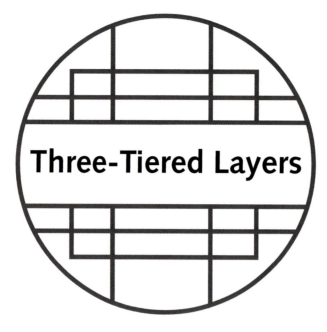

**Three-Tiered Layers**

*Using a three-tiered layering technique,
a short, sexy, asymmetric look is created*

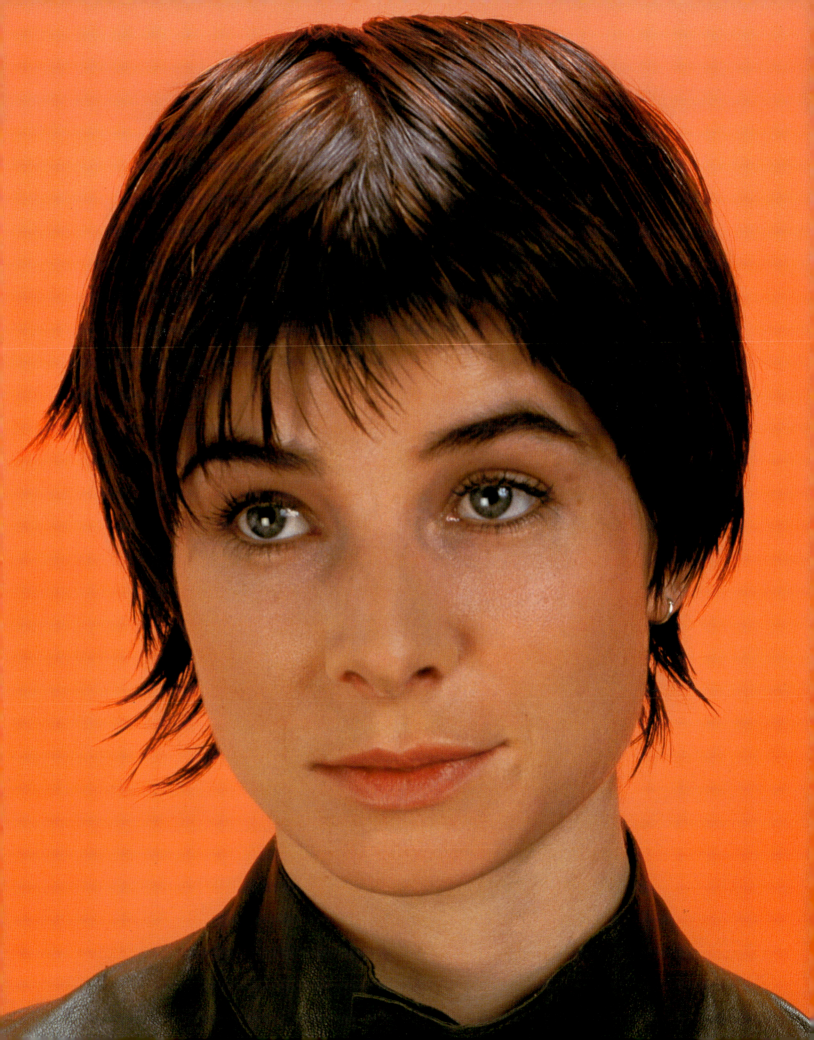

# Cutting

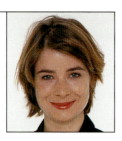

*The model's hair had been cut about four months previously. After a discussion we decided to go for a layered, textured look that would look easy, natural and totally modern.*

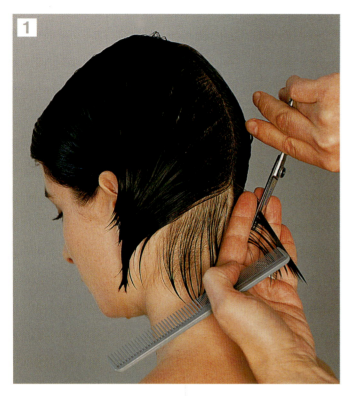

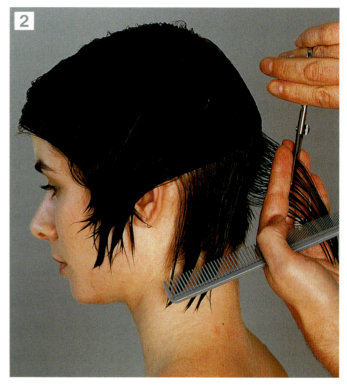

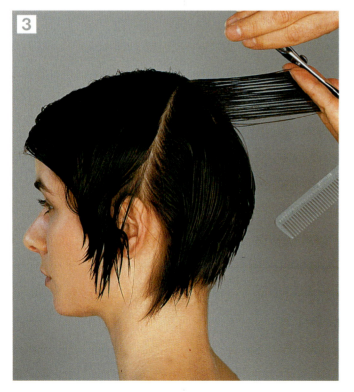

**1** Section out the first panel approximately 3 cm deep and parallel to the hairline. Take all your sections in this panel to finger width.

**2** Bring down the next panel approximately 3 cm deep. Start a completely new line; the length of the hair should correspond to cover the natural hairline.

**3** Bring down the next panel crown to the top of the ear and begin a new line. The longest length of the section should hang over the occipital bone.

Note: You have created three separate tiers of hair through the back of the head and although they do not technically check, they aesthetically balance, creating an open texture to the hair.

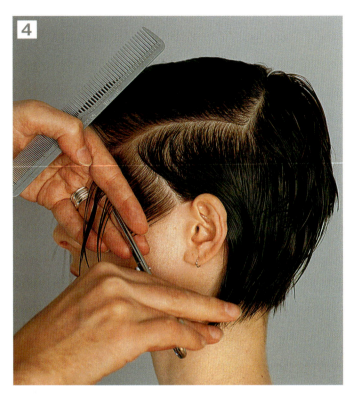

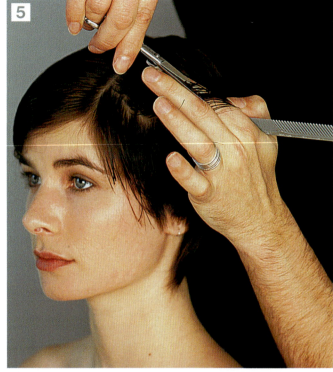

**4** Take a panel from the temple, cutting a section parallel to the hairline, work this line through to the back until the hair runs out.

**5** Take your next panel and cut your section to allow the outside length to be long enough to cover the hairline.

**6** Continue same technique on the other side creating an asymmetry to the fringe.

The hair is now ready for colouring.

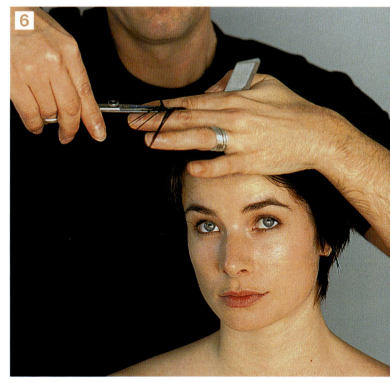

# Colouring

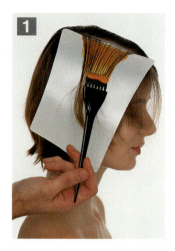
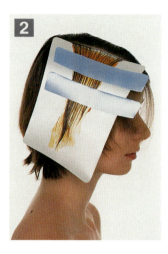
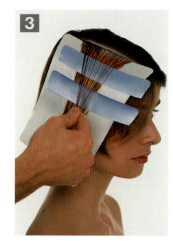
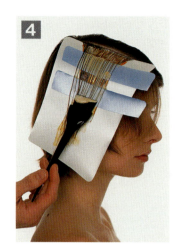

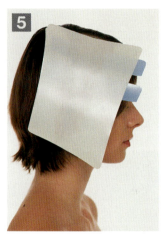
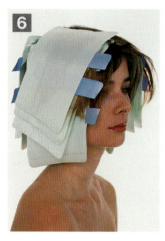
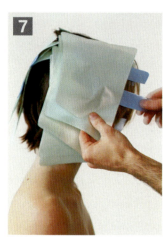

**1** A fine section is taken from the parting and placed on a Creative Colour Wrap and coloured using Wella Koleston Perfect 88/43 Vibrant Celtic Copper mixed with 6% Wella Welloxon Perfect Creme Developer

**2** Two pre-cut pieces of Creative Colour Wrap are then placed horizontally across the coloured section. Note that these pieces are allowed to protrude from the main Colour Wrap.

**3 + 4** A fine section from above is now placed on top of the Colour Wrap. This piece is then coloured using Wella Koleston Perfect 7/75 Warm Heather mixed with 6% Wella Welloxon Perfect Creme Developer from roots to ends.

**5** A Creative Colour Wrap is laid on top to seal.

**6** Continue working this technique through the top sections.

**7** Colour is now allowed to process for half the normal development time. Then the pre-cut Colour Wrap sections are slid out to allow colours to merge/fuse together. The colour is then allowed to process the remainder of the development time. When finished, shampoo and condition as normal.

# Finished Look

Dry the hair with Wella SP Styling Spray Lotion and finish with Wella SP Mould & Shine Creme.

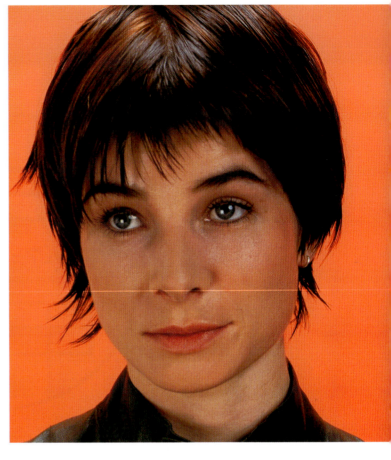

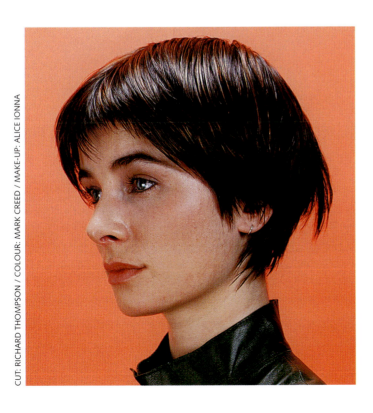

## Products used

Wella Koleston Perfect:
88/43 Vibrant Celtic Copper
7/75 Warm Heather

6% Wella Welloxon
Perfect Creme Developer

Wella SP Styling Spray Lotion

Wella SP Mould & Shine Creme

55

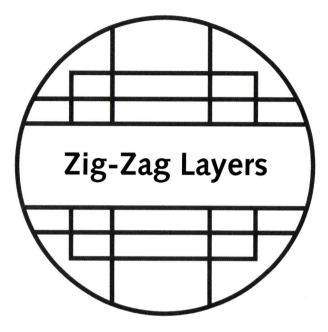

## Zig-Zag Layers

*Max out the layers with a mis-matched texture worn dishevelled or with a polished finish*

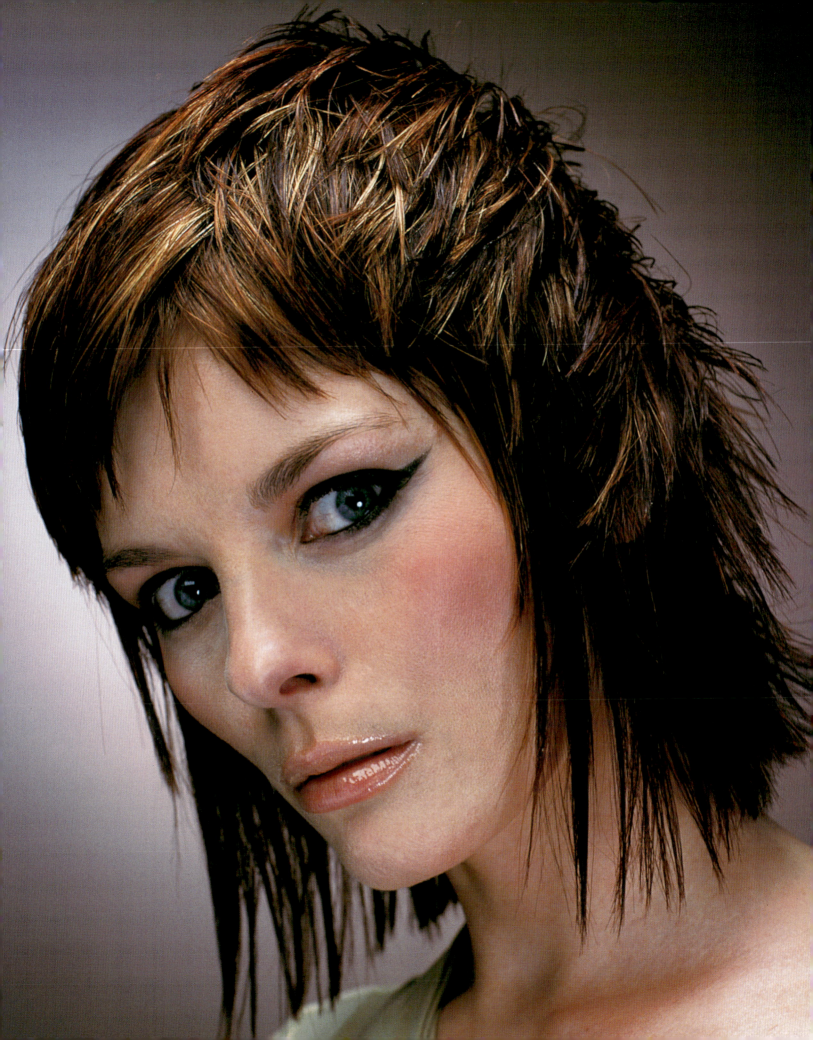

# Colouring

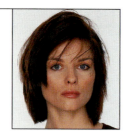

*Our model's hair was in a grown out-layered shape. She wanted a stronger modern look without losing her outline length. The colour was brown, golden shades were added to enhance the texture of the cut.*

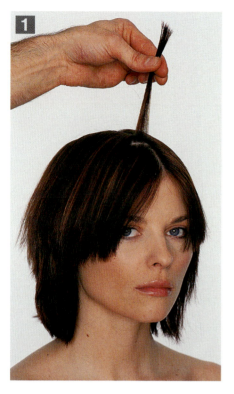

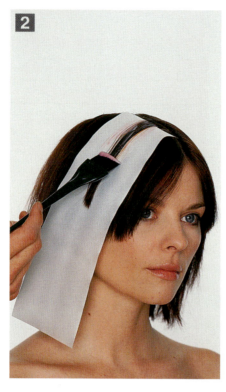

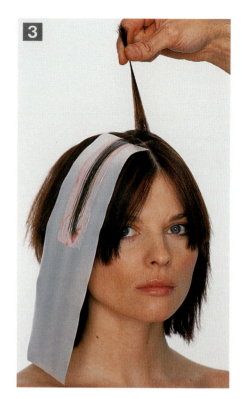

**1** Take a small triangular section from the parting.

**2** Place the section on a Colour Wrap and apply Wella Koleston Perfect 9/34 Soft Copper Gold and 9% Wella Welloxon Perfect Creme Developer.

**3** Take a triangular section from opposite side of parting.

**4** Place on a Colour Wrap and apply Wella Koleston Perfect 10/3 Lightest Golden Blonde and 9% Wella Welloxon Perfect Creme Developer.

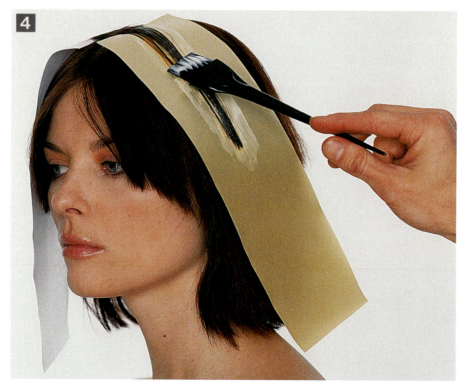

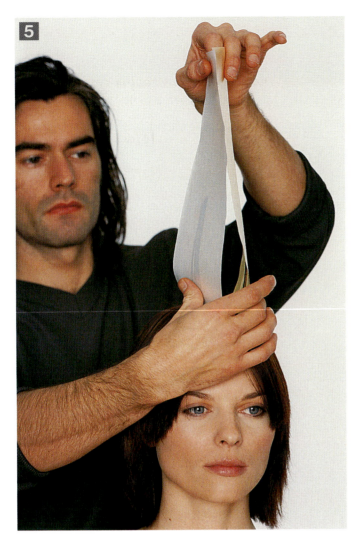

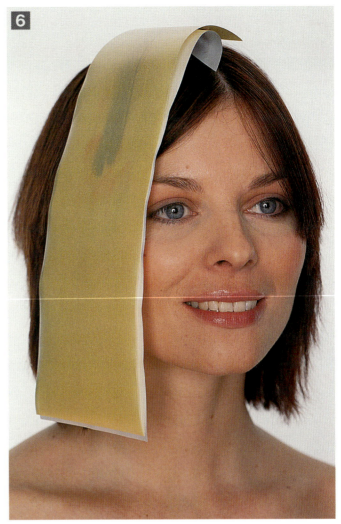

**5** Lift both Colour Wraps and seal fusing both colours together.

**6** Sealed Colour Wrap with the two triangular sections with the two chosen colours fused together.

**7** Continue this technique through the entire head missing fine sections out in between Colour Wraps.

Allow colour to process, then shampoo and condition as normal.

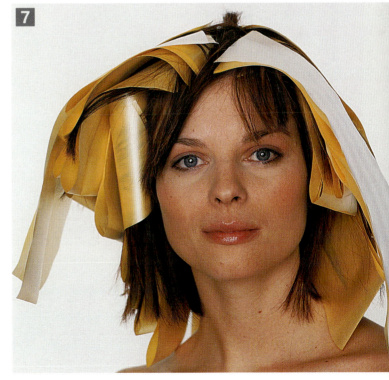

# Cutting

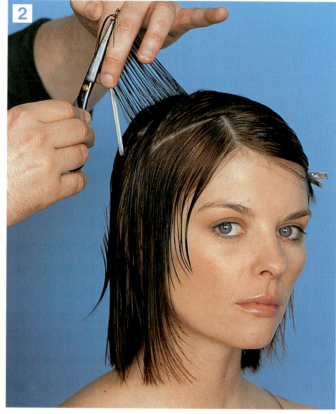

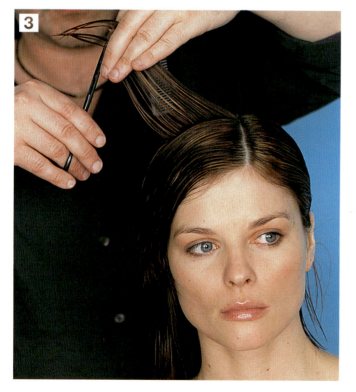

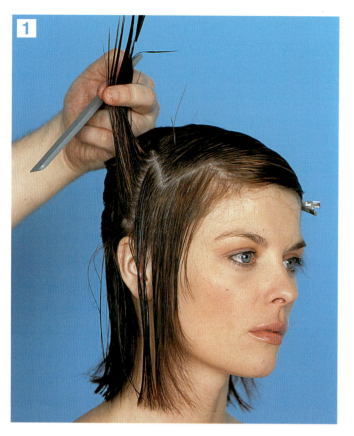

**1** Section out top panel using zig-zag sectioning through the sides.

Lift under panel sections vertically and texturise by cutting long V-sections into the ends. Work around the head in this way on all underneath panels.

**2** Take down top panel and begin a new line that checks aesthetically, but not technically, with the previously cut under sections.

**3** Continue line over central partings.

Repeat on opposite side.

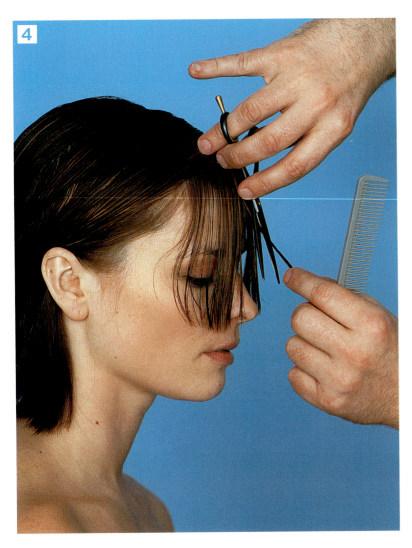

**4** Slice-cut fringe area to desired length.

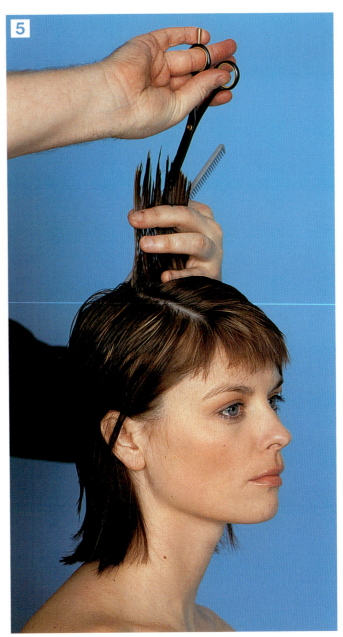

**5** Cut texture into top panel by cutting long deep V-sections into lengths.

# Finished Look

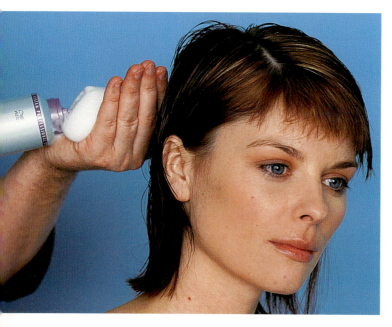

Wella SP Texturising Mousse was applied.

Hair was dried and finished with Wella SP Sculpting Gel for tough separation of texture.

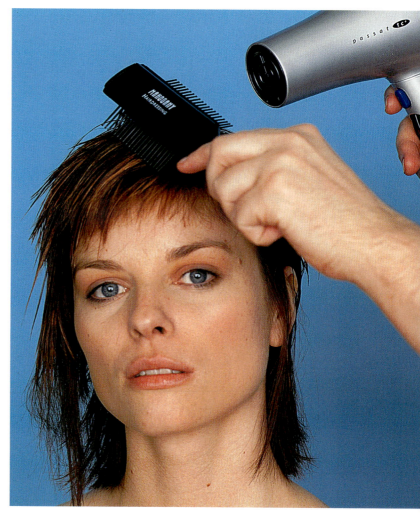

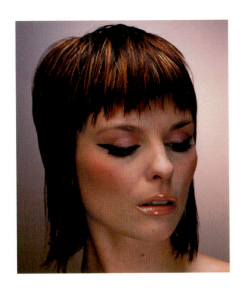
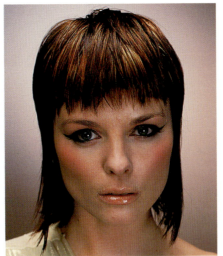
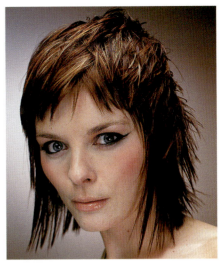

## Products used

Wella Koleston Perfect:
    9/34 Soft Copper Gold
    10/3 Lightest Golden Blonde

9% Wella Welloxon
Perfect Creme Developer

Wella SP Texturising Mousse

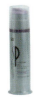

Wella SP Sculpting Gel

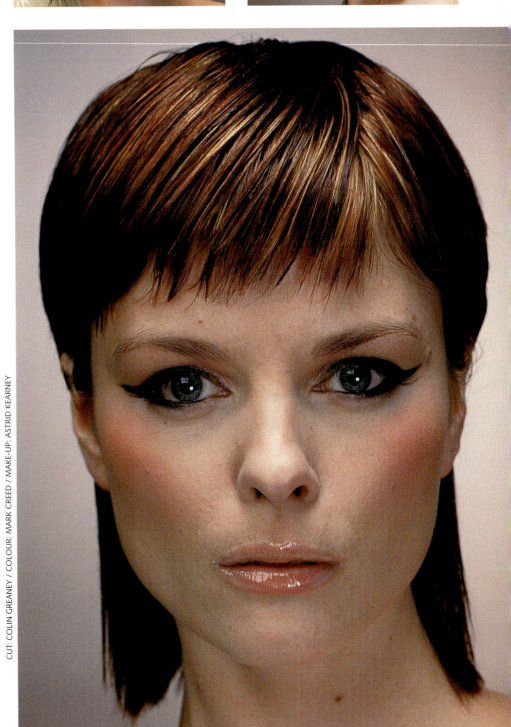

CUT: COLIN GREANEY / COLOUR: MARK CREED / MAKE-UP: ASTRID KEARNEY

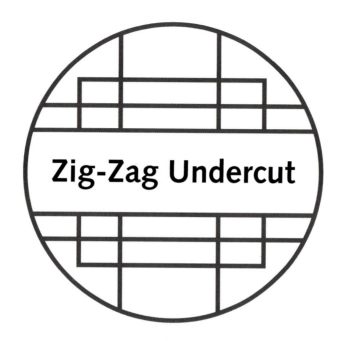

**Zig-Zag Undercut**

By using zig-zag sections and disconnecting the top lengths of hair a modern, short, textured cut is created

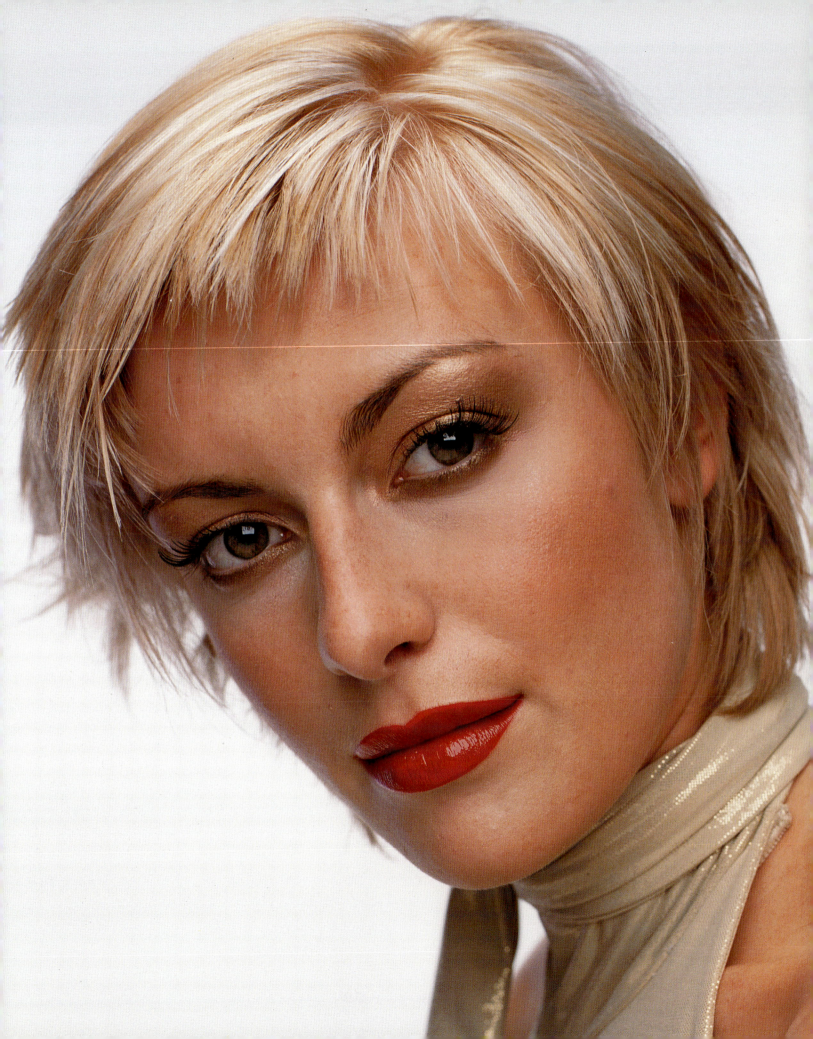

# Colouring

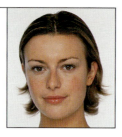

*Our model has grown out a short hair cut.*
*She wants to be blonde and have a funkier look.*

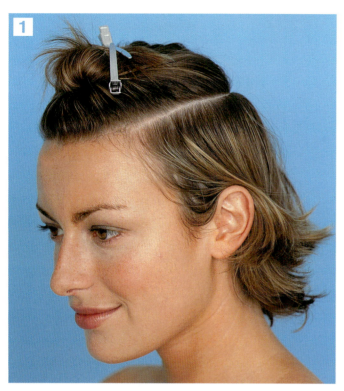

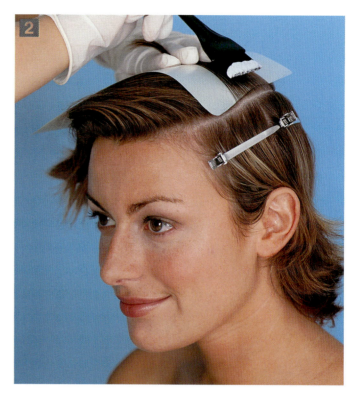

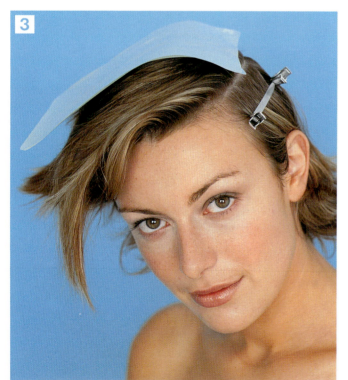

**1** Section the top panel from the under panel.

**2** Take the first slice using Creative Colour Wraps. Work diagonally across the head and apply Wella Blondor Special with 6% Wella Welloxon Perfect Creme Developer.

**3** Seal with a second Creative Colour Wrap.

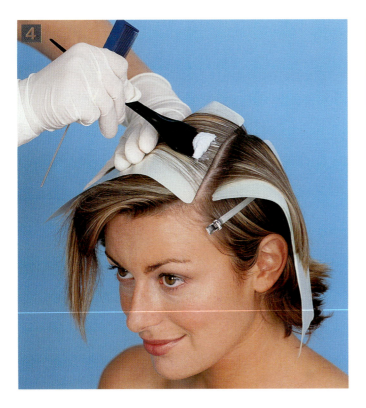

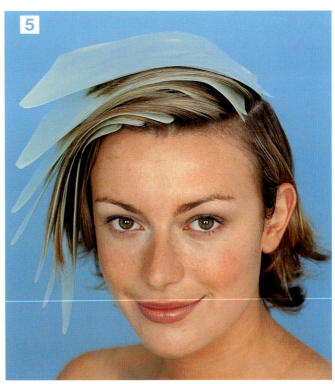

**4** Note how the shape of the Creative Colour Wraps fit the head shape.

**5** All slices are now in place.

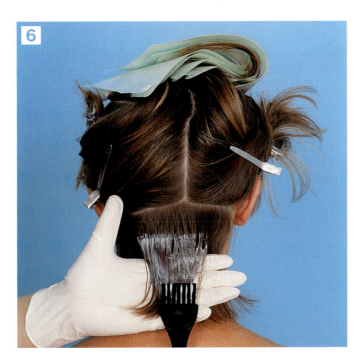

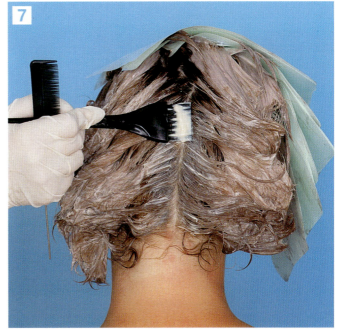

**6** Apply Wella Koleston Perfect 12/16 Special Soft Ash mixed with 12% Wella Welloxon Perfect Creme Developer to mid-lengths and ends as quickly as possible.

**7** Once the mid-lengths and ends have processed apply Wella Koleston Perfect 12/16 Special Soft Ash with 12% Wella Welloxon Perfect Creme Developer to the roots. Leave to process. When the correct colour is achieved, spritz the bleach and wipe from the packets. Shampoo and condition as normal.

# Cutting

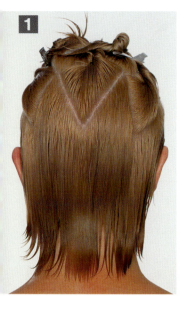

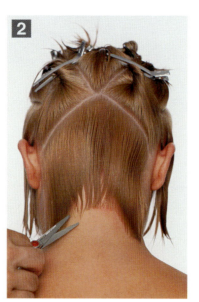

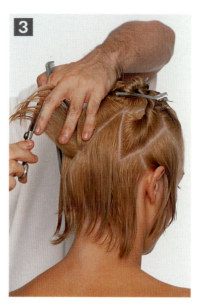

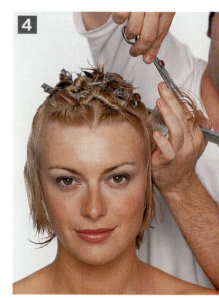

**1** Section the top panel away in a zig-zag pattern.

**2** Establish an inverted outline shape.

**3** Layer the under sections parallel to the head.

**4** Continue to layer all the under panel parallel to the head shape lifting the outline up to maintain the outline length.

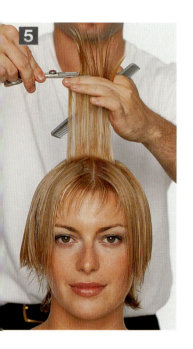

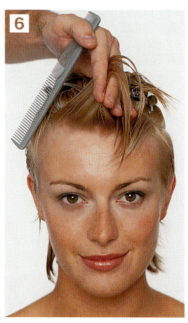

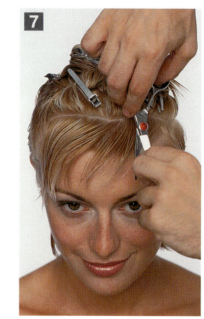

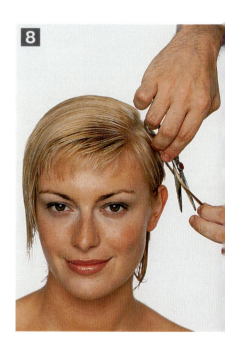

**5** Let down the top panel and start a new line. Layer across the top allowing the top lengths to overhang the under panel to a visually balanced length.

**6** Establish the length of the fringe. This length doesn't check in with the top hair.

**7** Texturise the fringe by slide cutting into lengths.

**8** Texturise the top lengths by slide cutting.

68

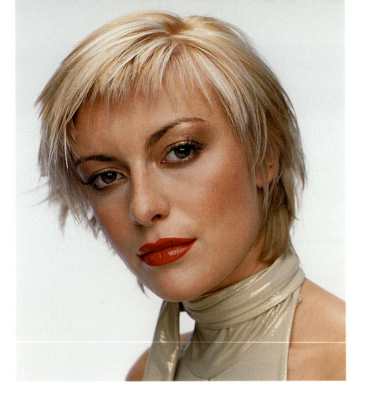

# Finished Look

The hair was dried and finished with Wella SP Ends Express.

## Products used

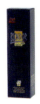

Wella Blondor Special Creme

6% Wella Welloxon Perfect Creme Developer

Wella Koleston Perfect: 12/16 Special Soft Ash

12% Wella Welloxon Perfect Creme Developer

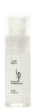

Wella SP Ends Express

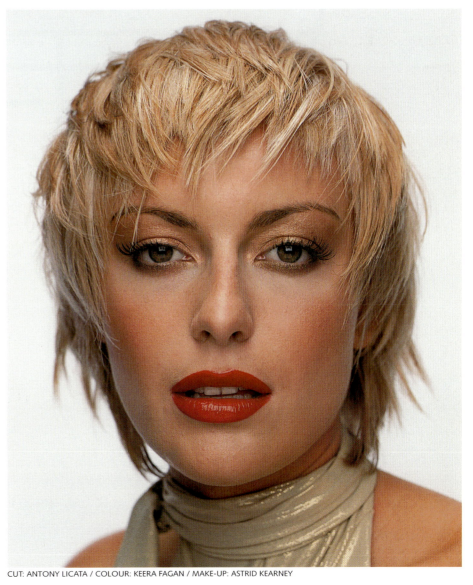

CUT: ANTONY LICATA / COLOUR: KEERA FAGAN / MAKE-UP: ASTRID KEARNEY

69

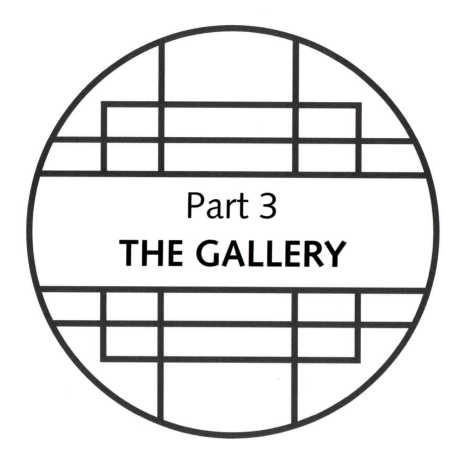

# Part 3
# THE GALLERY

*Looks created by the Mahogany Creative Team*
*as directives for modern classics*

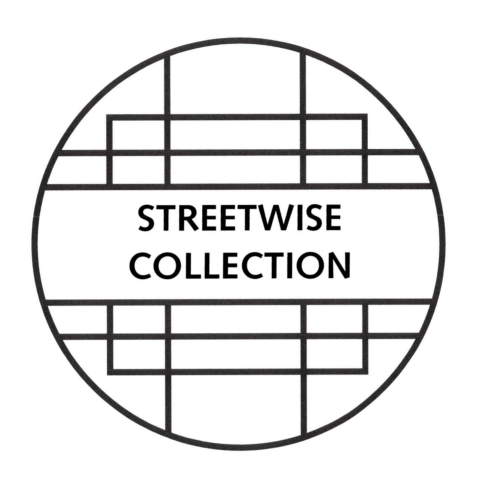

STREETWISE
COLLECTION

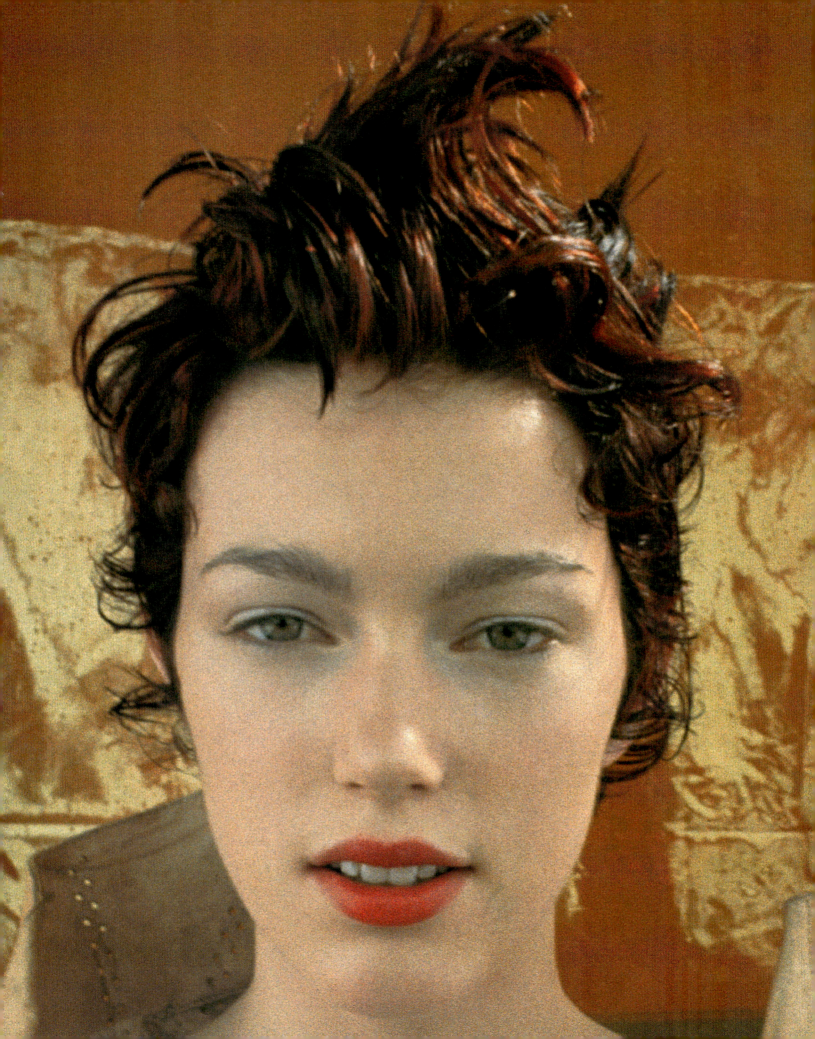

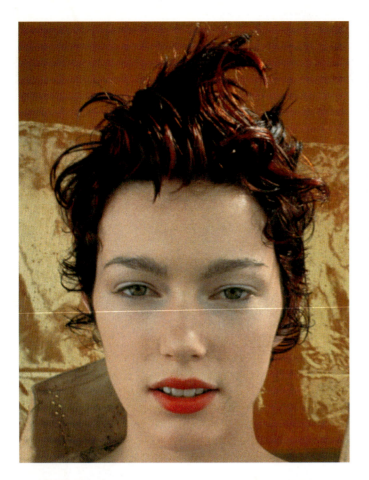
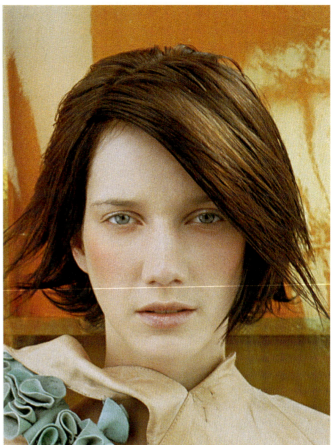
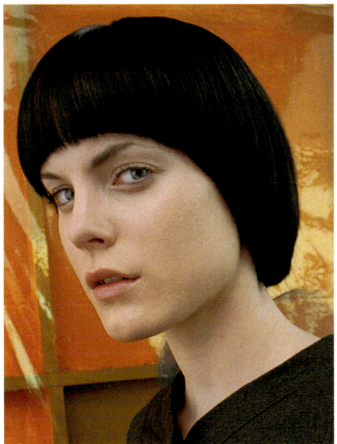
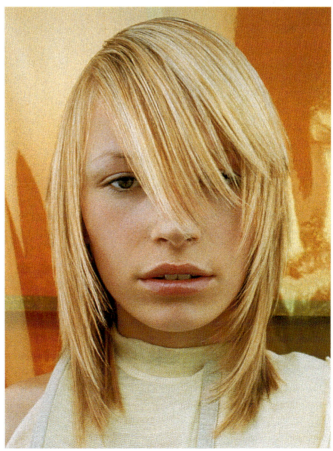

HAIR: CHARLIE HALE/ COLOUR: MARK CREED / PHOTOGRAPHY: ALBERTO BADALAMENTI / MAKE-UP SHARON IVES / CLOTHES BY JULIA CLANCEY / PRODUCTS: WELLA

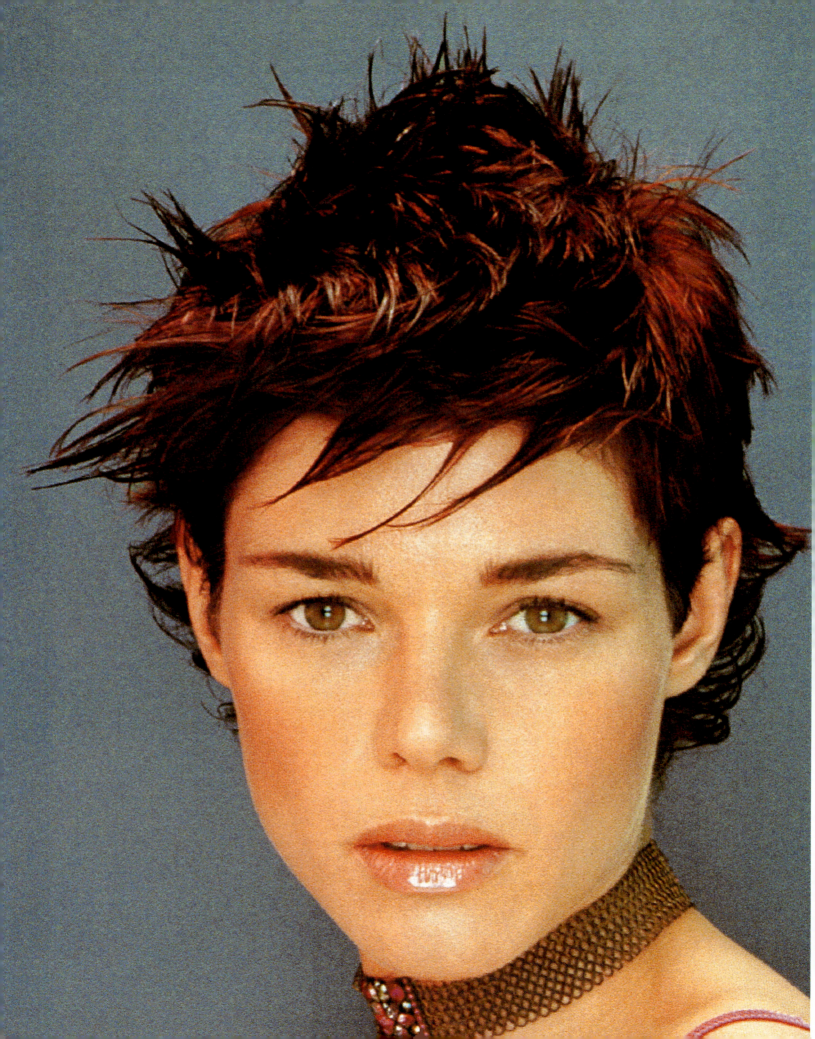

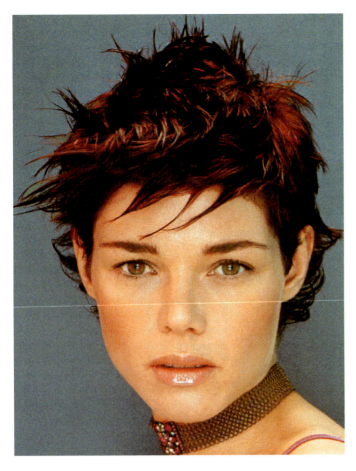
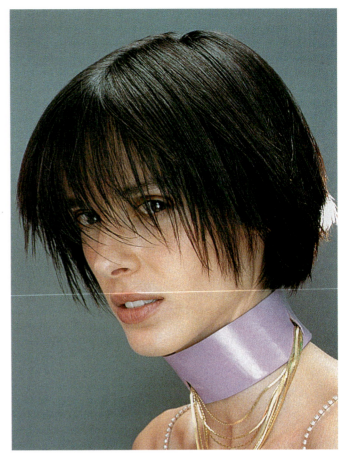
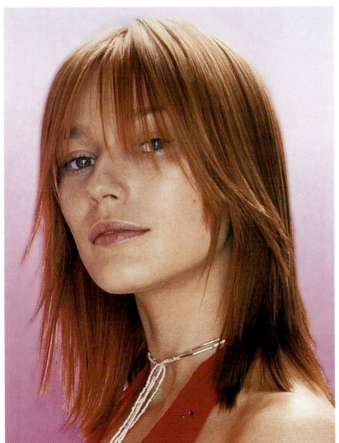
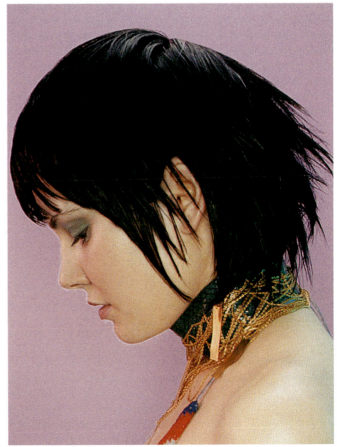

HAIR: ANTONY LICATA / PHOTOGRAPHY: ALBERTO BADALAMENTI / CLOTHES STYLING: JULIA CLANCEY / MAKE-UP: SHARON IVES / PRODUCTS: WELLA

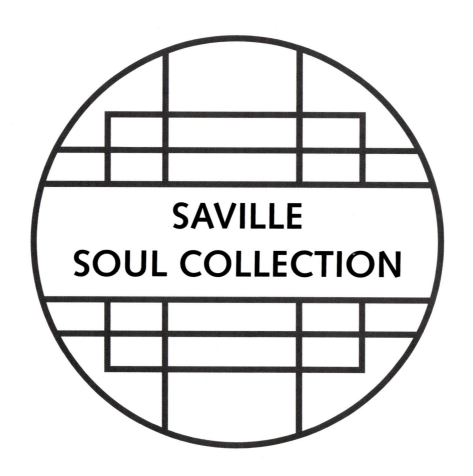

SAVILLE
SOUL COLLECTION

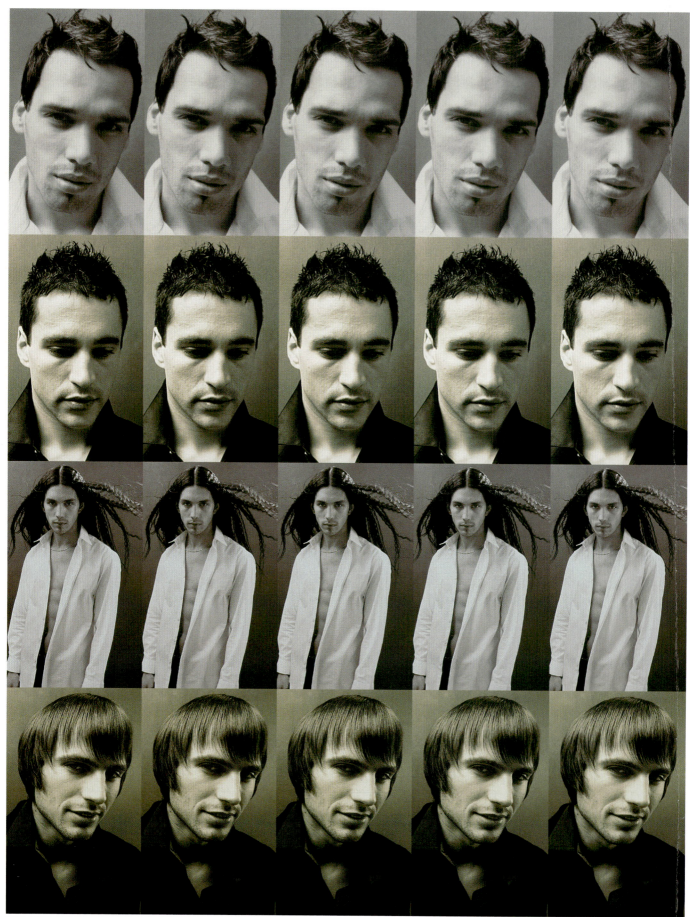

HAIR: ROBYN FENTON / PHOTOGRAPHY: ALBERTO BADALAMENTI / CLOTHES STYLING: JULIA CLANCEY / GROOMING: SHARON IVES / PRODUCTS: WELLA

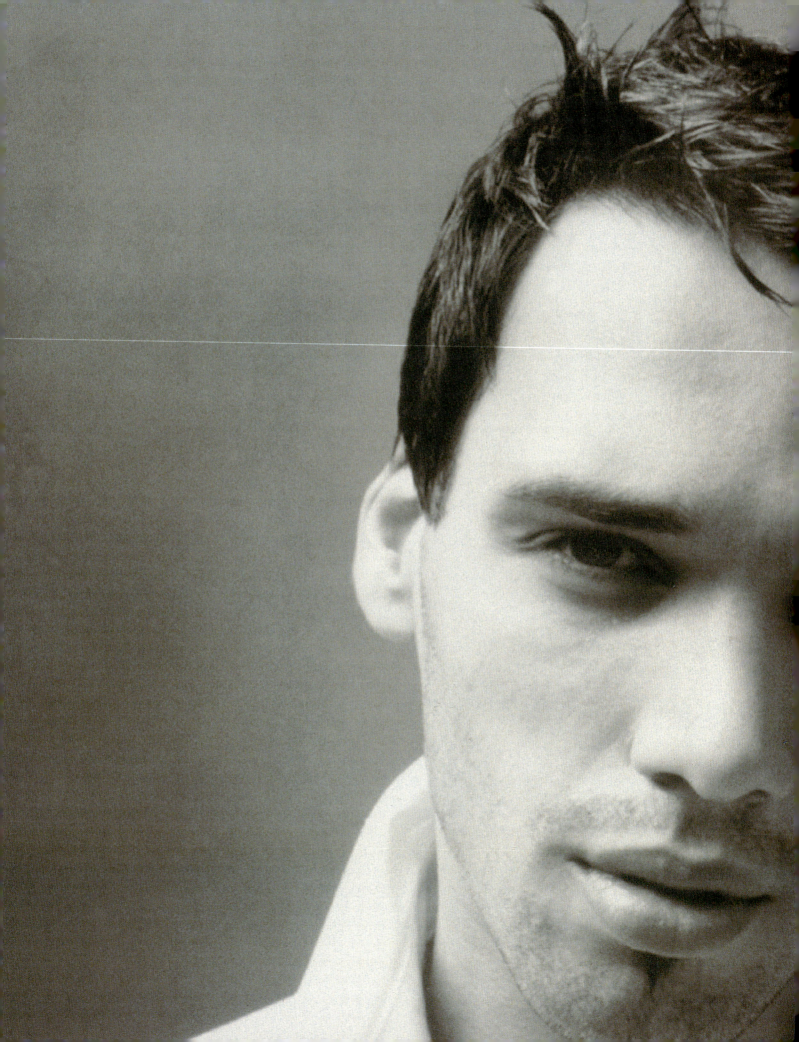

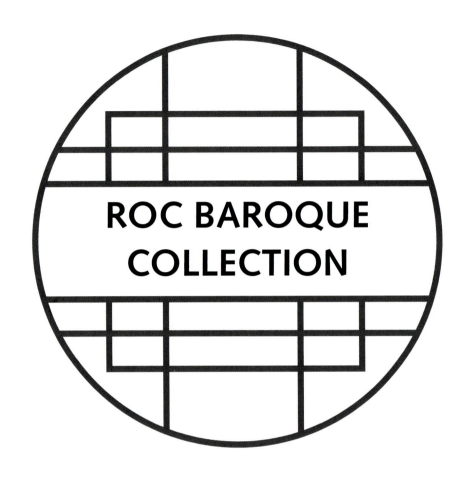

ROC BAROQUE
COLLECTION

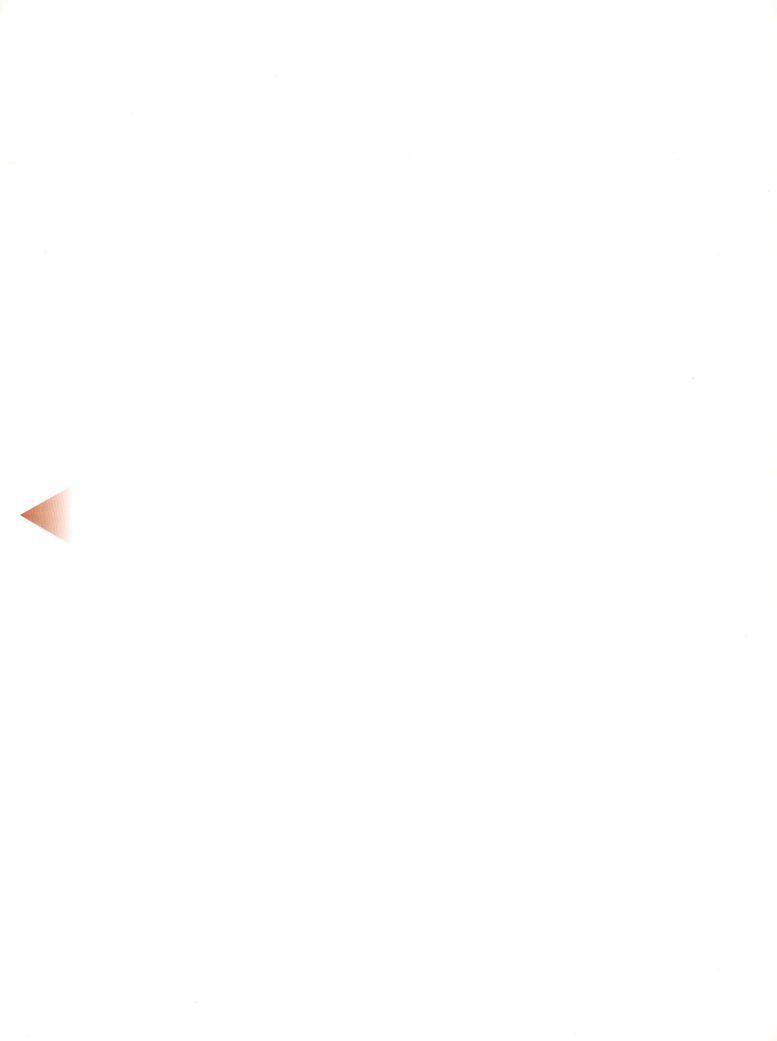

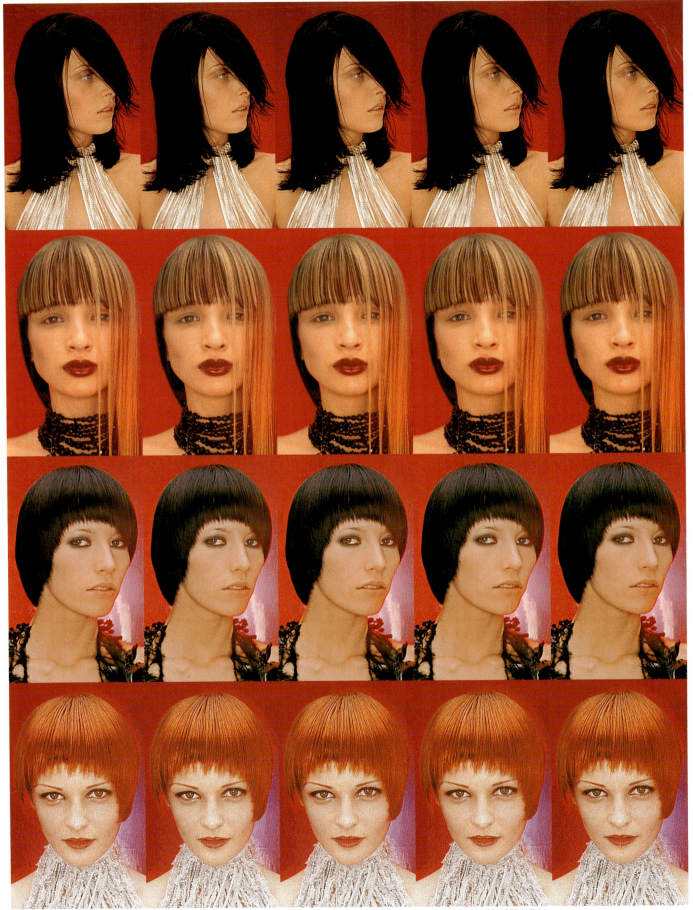

CUT: RICHARD THOMPSON / COLOUR: MARK CREED / PHOTOGRAPHY: ALBERTO BADALAMENTI / CLOTHES: JULIA CLANCEY / PRODUCTS: WELLA

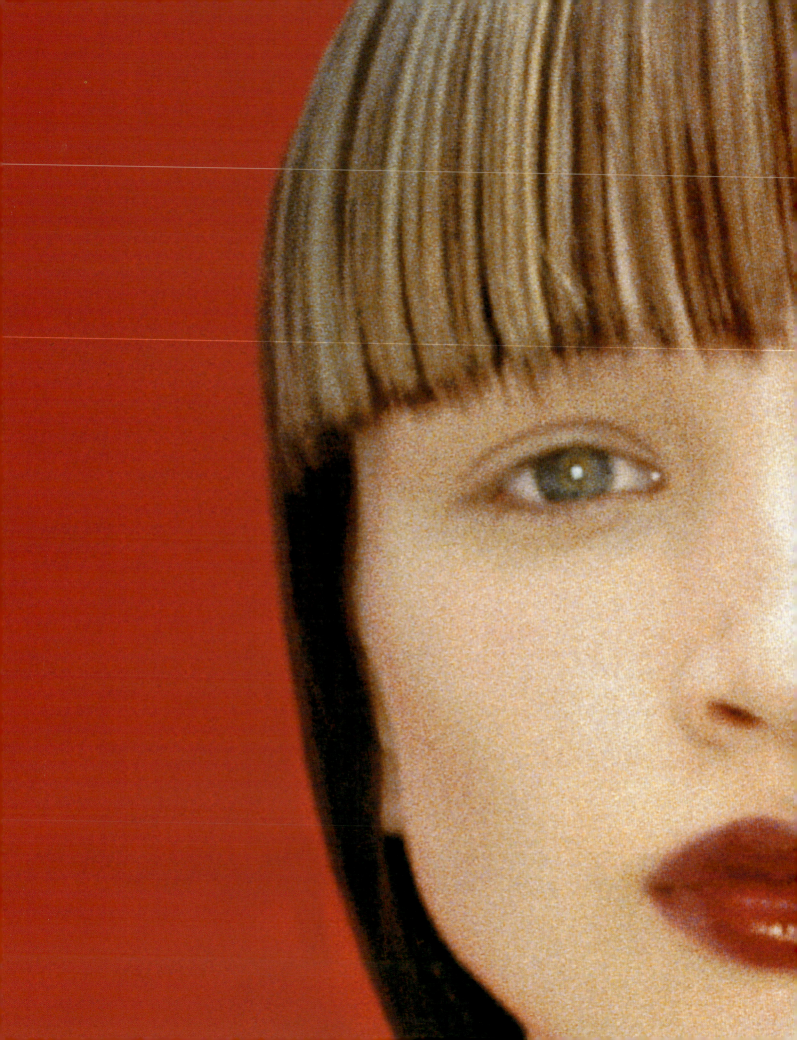

URBAN ETHNICITY
COLLECTION

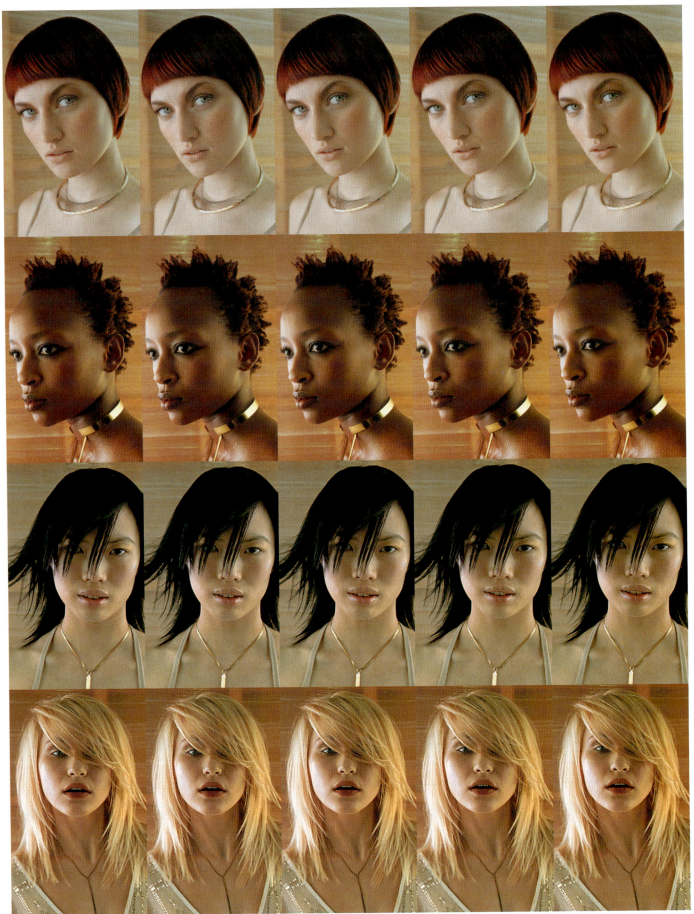

CUT: COLIN GREANEY / PHOTOGRAPHY: ALBERTO BADALAMENTI / CLOTHES STYLING: JULIA CLANCEY / MAKE-UP: SHARON IVES / PRODUCTS: WELLA

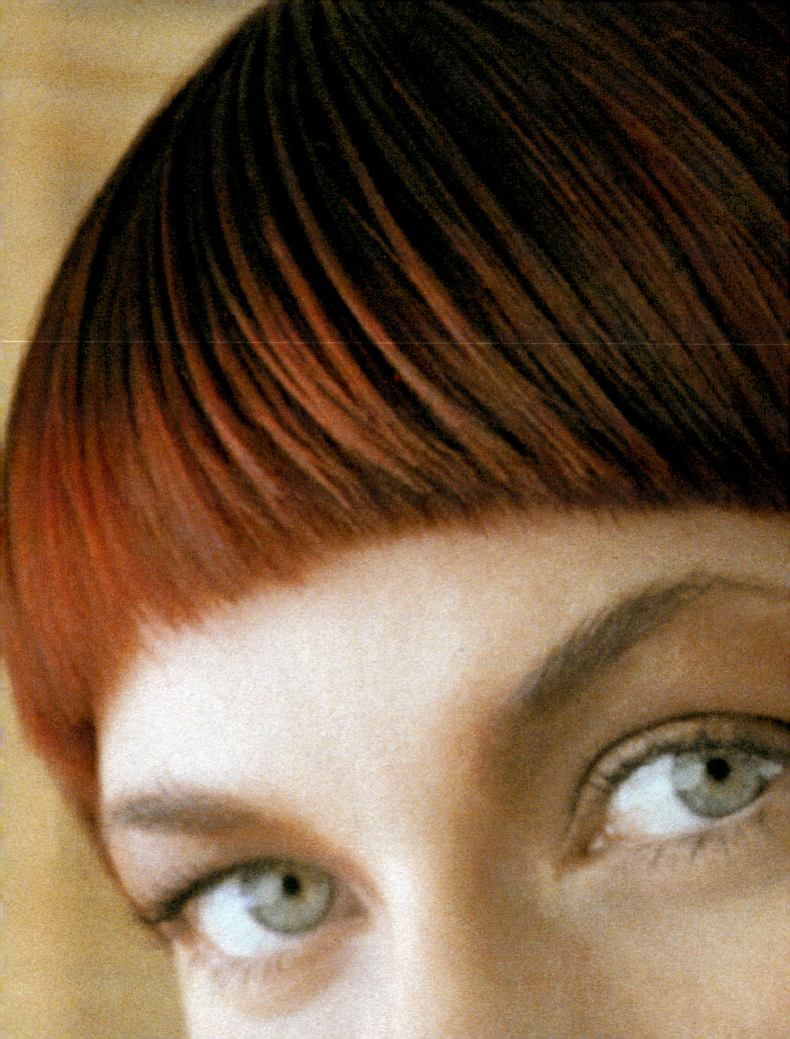

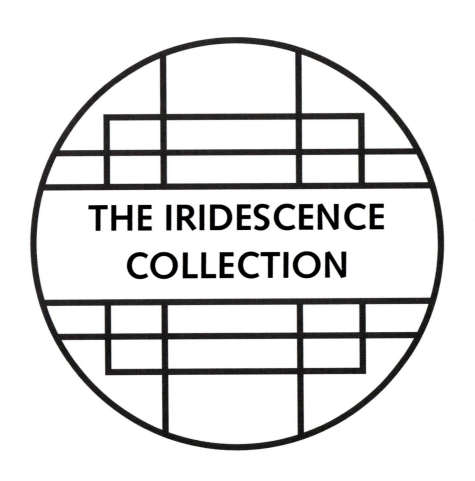

THE IRIDESCENCE
COLLECTION

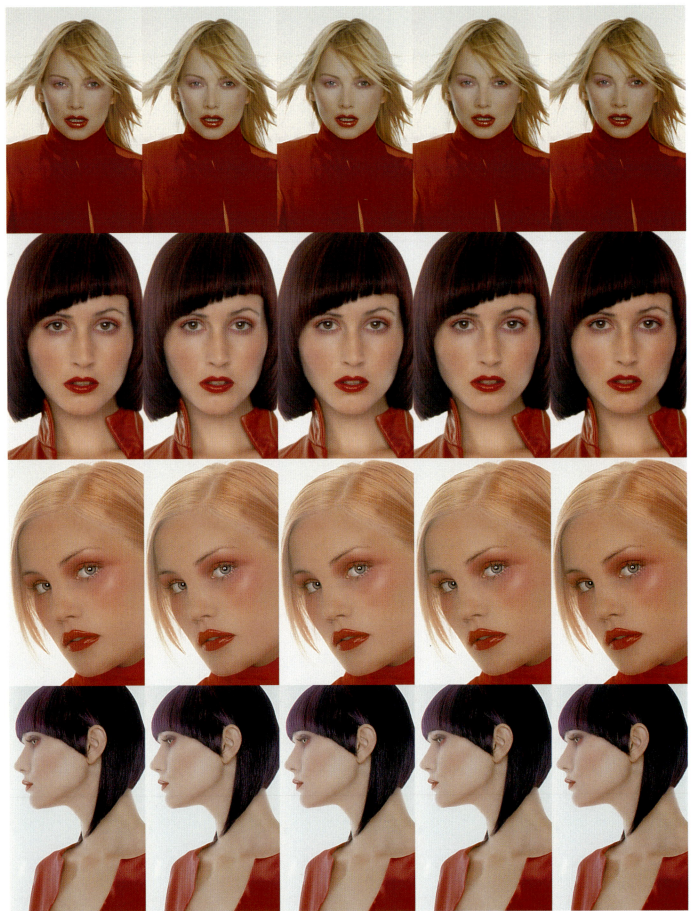

CUT: RICHARD THOMPSON & COLIN GREANEY / COLOUR: MARK CREED / PHOTOGRAPHY: MIKE DIVER / CLOTHES : JULIA CLANCEY / MAKE-UP: ASTRID KEARNEY / PRODUCTS: WELLA

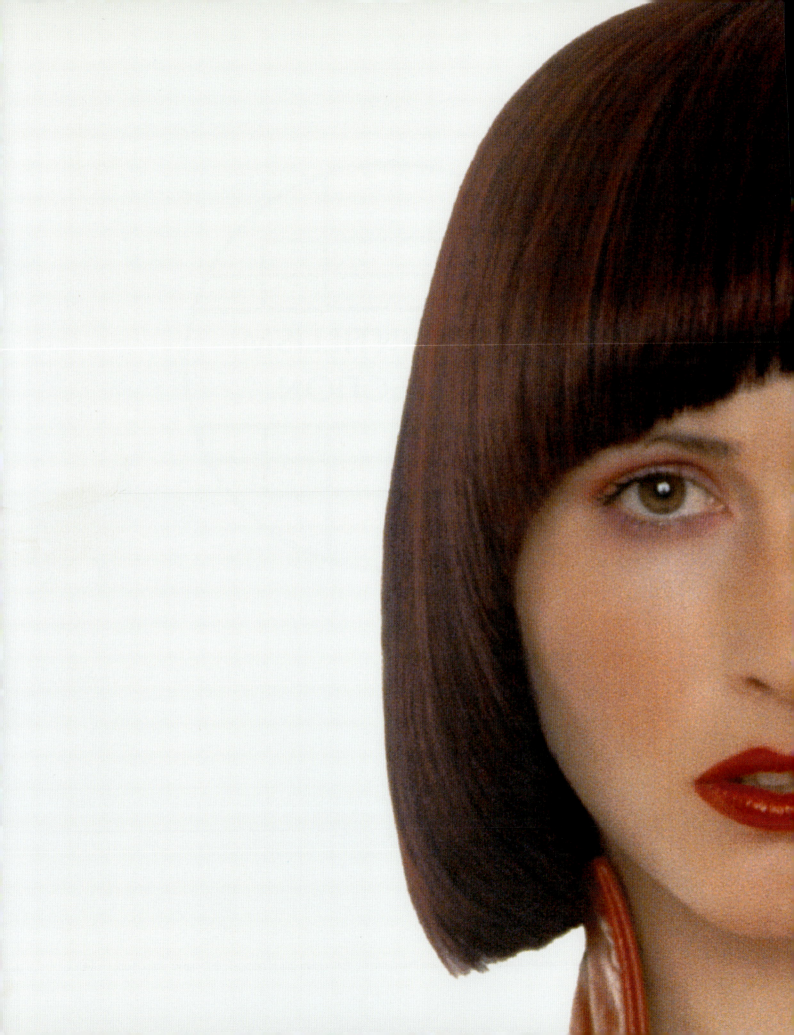

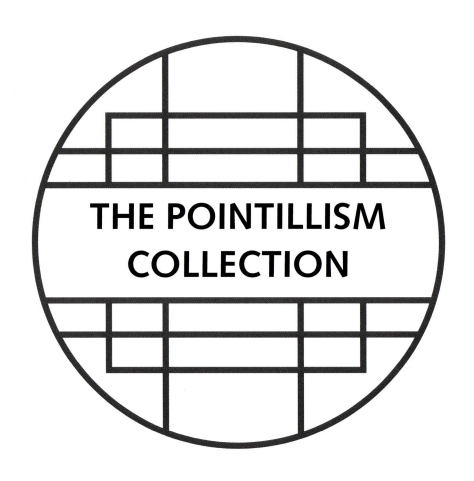

THE POINTILLISM
COLLECTION

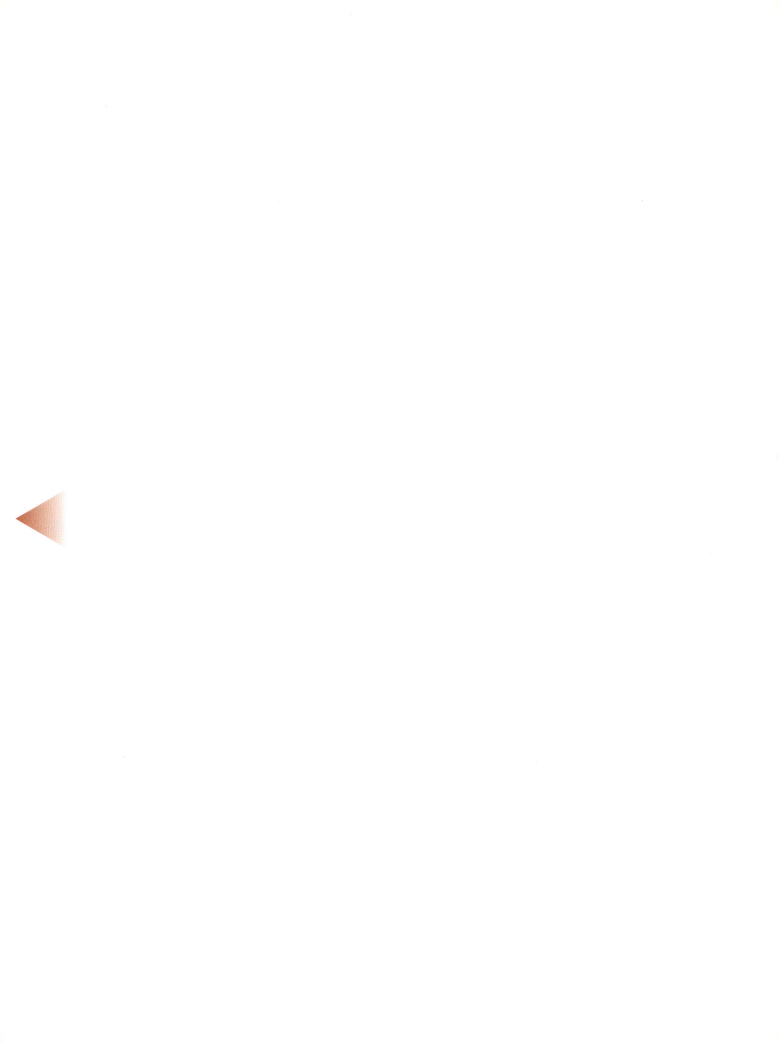

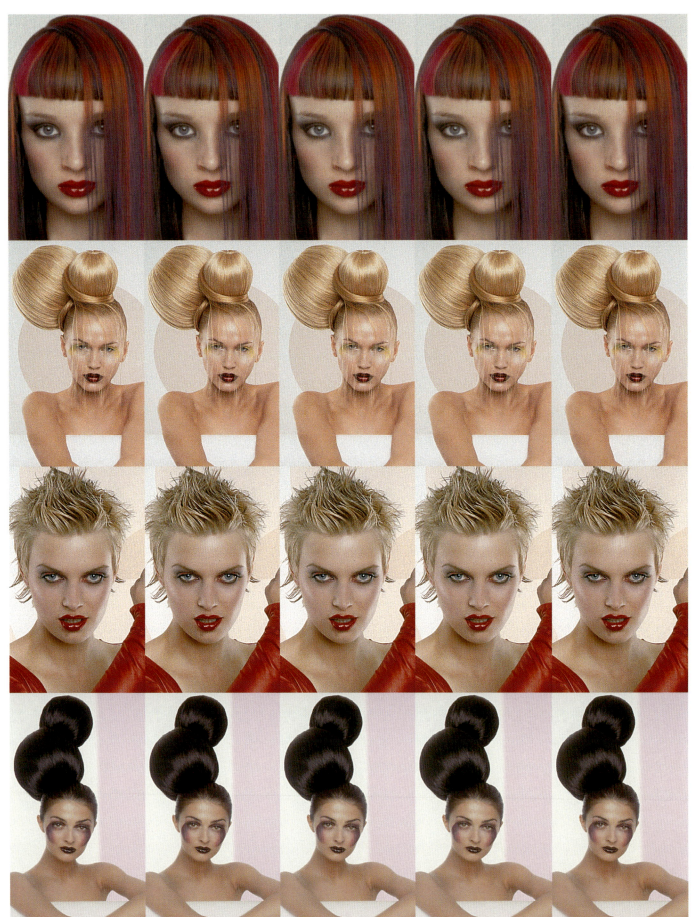

HAIR: RICHARD THOMPSON / COLOUR: MARK CREED / PHOTOGRAPHY: MIKE DIVER / CLOTHES : JULIA CLANCEY / MAKE-UP: ASTRID KEARNEY / PRODUCTS: WELLA

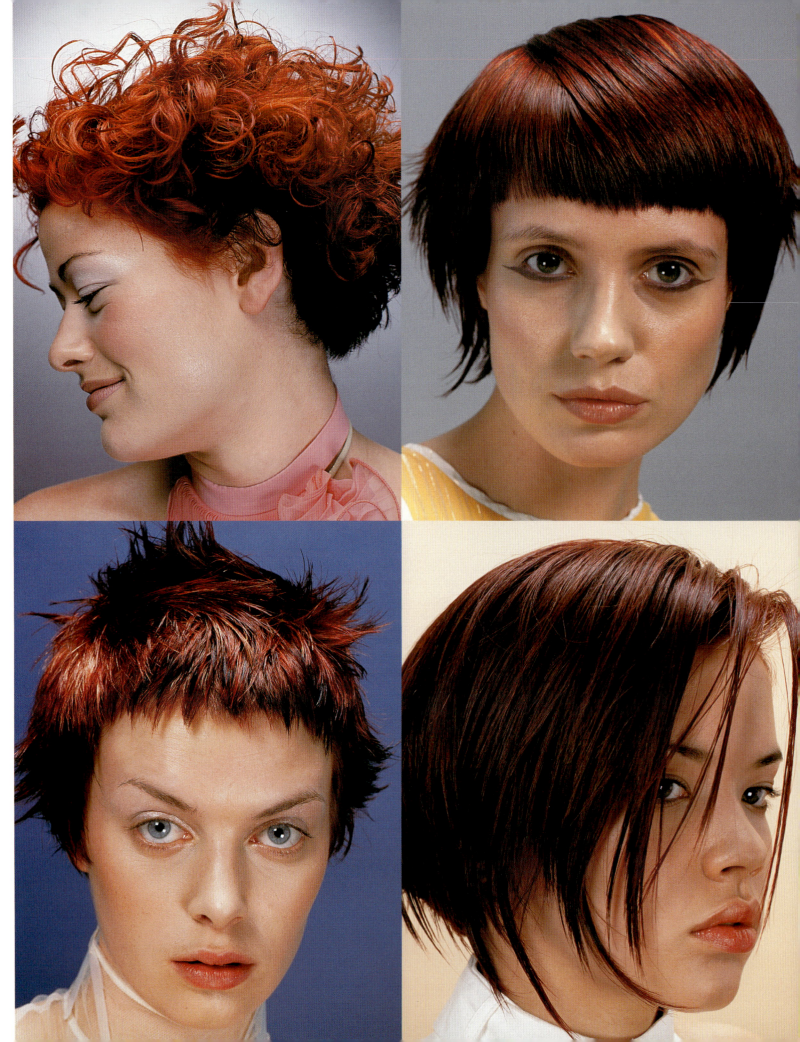

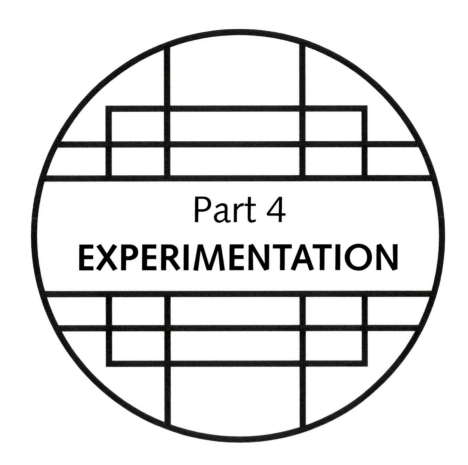

# Part 4
# EXPERIMENTATION

*Combine layering, graduation and undercutting.*
*Create contemporary cut and colour images.*

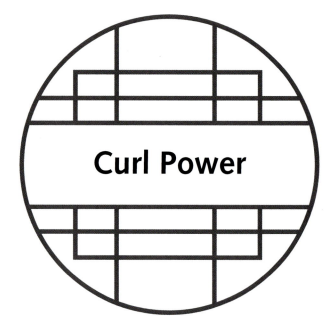

# Curl Power

*Maintaining control in the outline,*
*set free the internal curl*

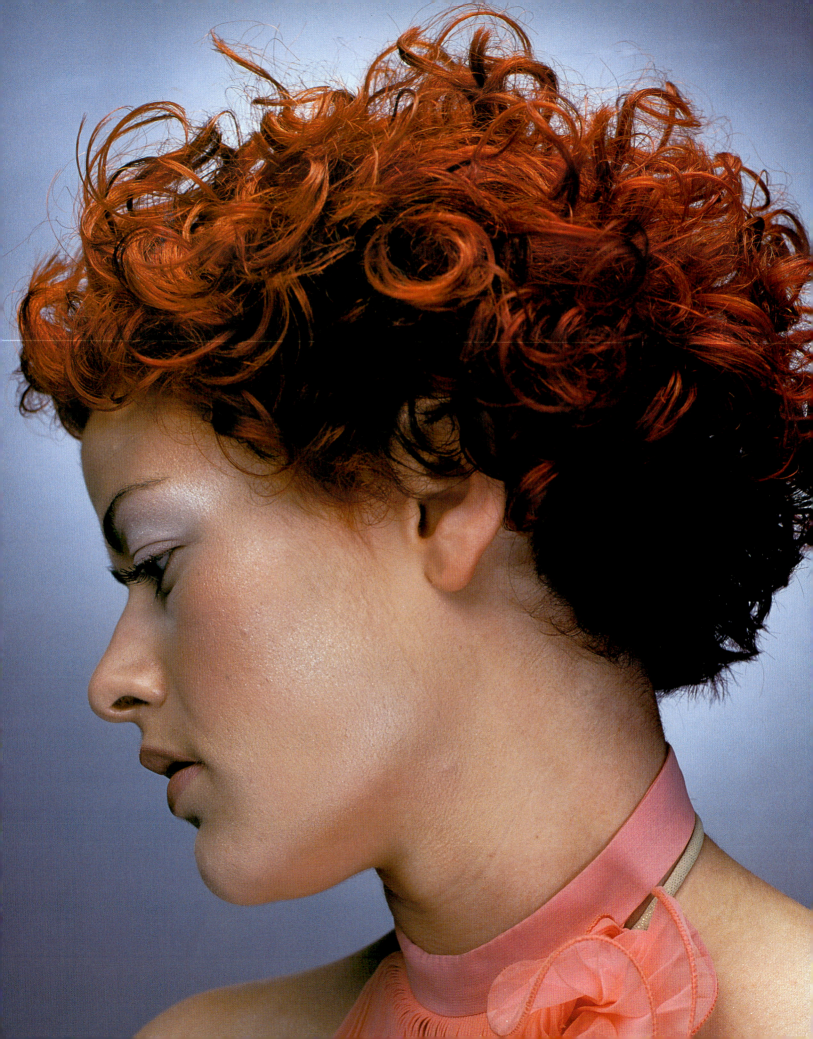

# Cutting

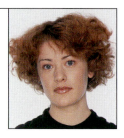

*Our model's hair is naturally curly and has grown out from a short, layered shape. She wants the colour to be brighter with a cut that will use her naturally curly hair.*

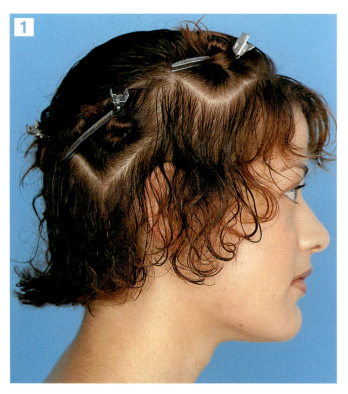

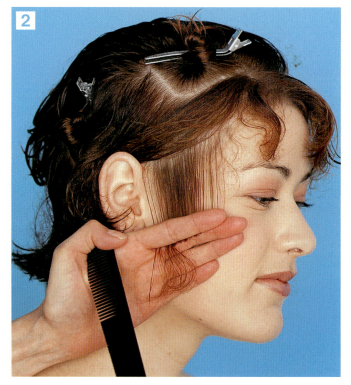

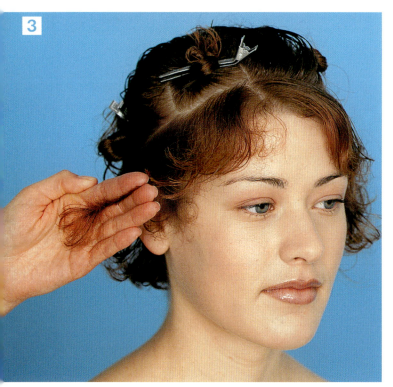

**1** Section hair in a zig-zag pattern.

**2** Cut a line from the cheekbone to the base of the ear.

**3** Lift hair to 45 degrees from the head using horizontal graduation techniques.

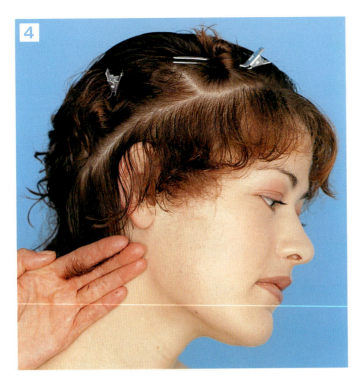

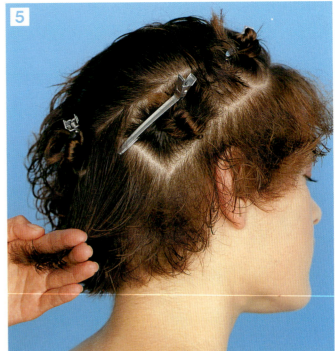

**4** Continue to nape.

**5** Horizontally graduate through the back lifting hair to 45 degrees from the head.
Note: When using the horizontal graduation technique ensure the head remains in the same position otherwise an unbalanced effect can be created.

**6** Take down the top panel and cut a square line across the top. Do not check in with the underneath panel.

**7** Cut an arc-shaped fringe. The centre of the fringe should be shorter.

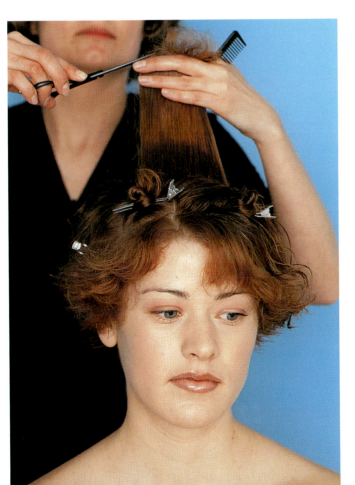

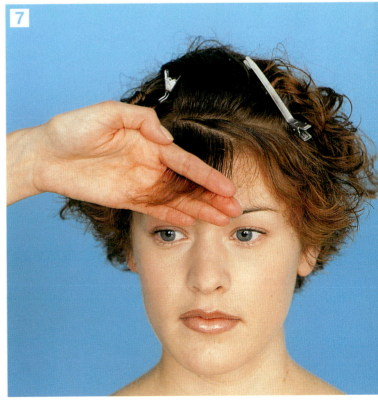

# Colouring

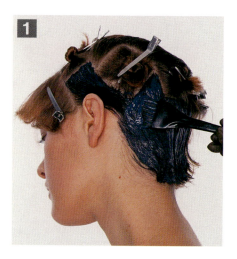

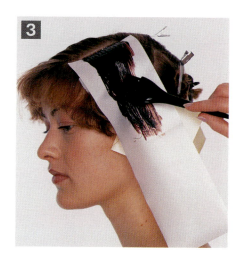

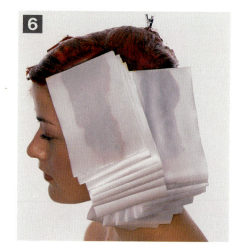

**1** Section hair into the original zig-zag pattern. Take two square panels within the top panel.
Apply colour to underneath panels using Wella Koleston Perfect 3/66 Deep Damson and 6% Wella Welloxon Perfect Creme Developer.

**2** Mask off this colour using Colour Wraps.

**3** Take down the two top square panels dividing them into slices and place in Colour Wraps alternating between Wella Koleston Perfect 8/4 Sunset Red, Wella Koleston Perfect 8/45 Rosso Red colour and 6% Wella WelloxonPerfect Creme Developer.

**4** Finished application of square panels.

**5** Apply Wella Koleston Perfect 77/44 Vibrant Flame Red and 6% Wella Welloxon Perfect Creme Developer to the remaining top panel.

**6** When finished, allow to process, then shampoo and condition as normal.

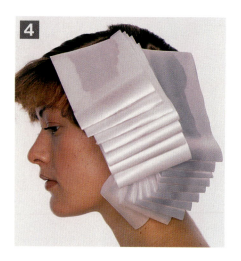

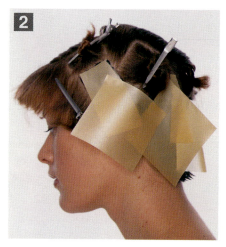

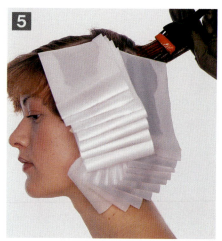

# Finished Look

The hair is dried using Wella SP Styling Spray Lotion and finished using Wella SP Mould & Shine Creme.

## Products used

Wella Koleston Perfect:
  3/66 Deep Damson
  8/4 Sunset Red
  8/45 Rosso Red
  77/44 Vibrant Flame Red

6% Wella Welloxon Perfect Creme Developer

Wella SP Styling Spray Lotion

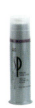

Wella SP Mould & Shine Creme

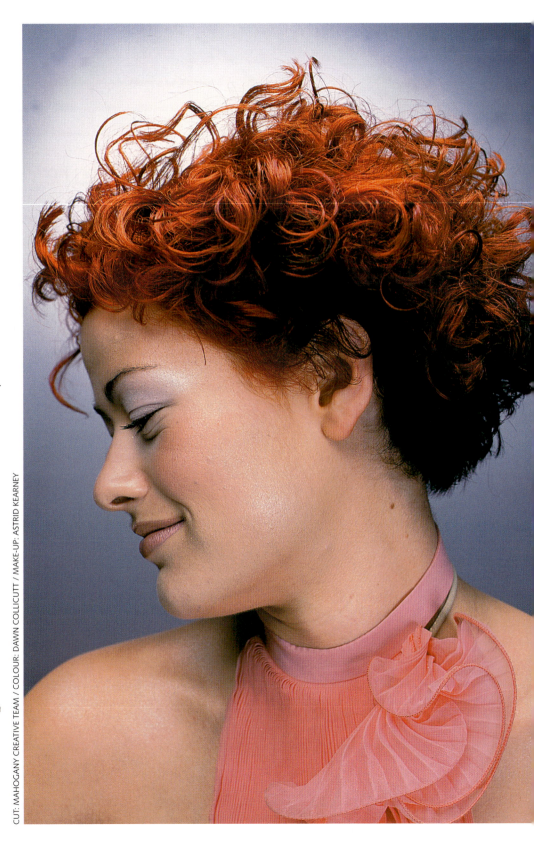

CUT: MAHOGANY CREATIVE TEAM / COLOUR: DAWN COLLICUTT / MAKE-UP: ASTRID KEARNEY

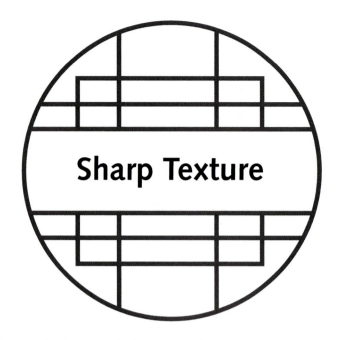

**Sharp Texture**

*A long V-section cutting technique combined with a short sharp fringe creates an ultra modern look*

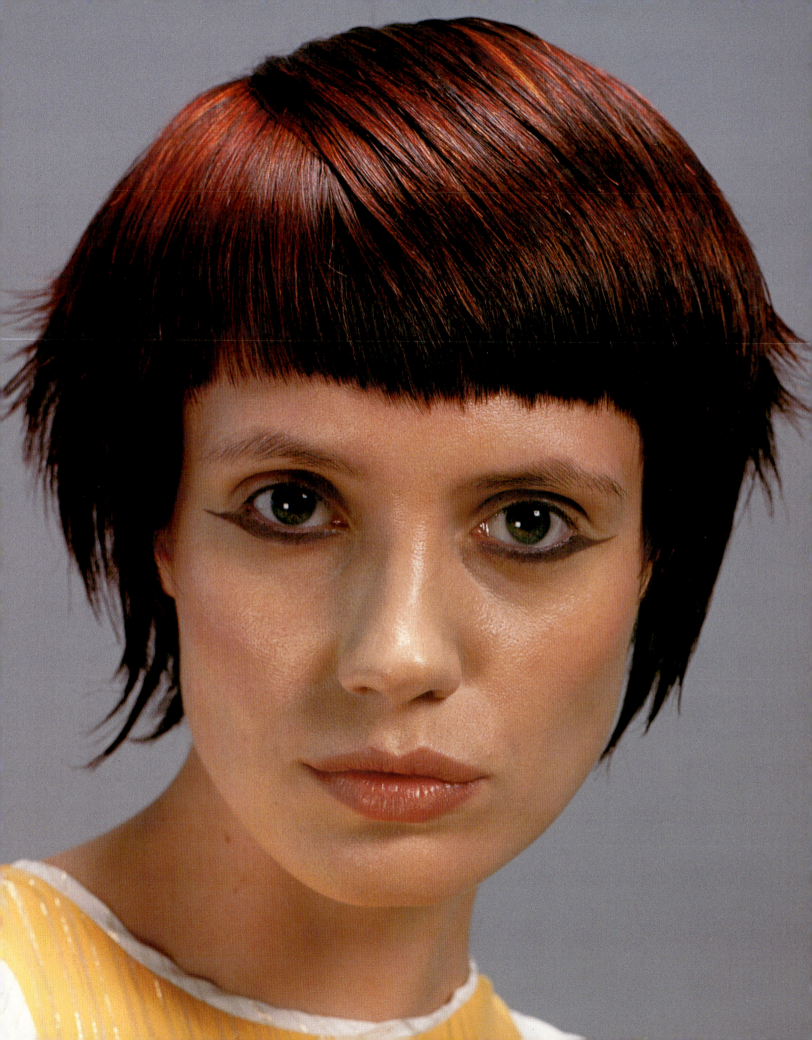

# Cutting

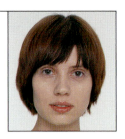

*The model's hair had been cut six weeks previously for another photo shoot. After consultation, it was established she wanted a stronger red colour and a narrower shape with shorter fringe. Her natural colour is 6/0 Dark Blonde and has been tinted using a hazel-toned colour, which has a 3 cm regrowth.*

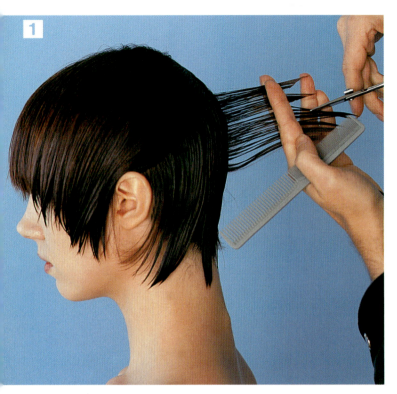

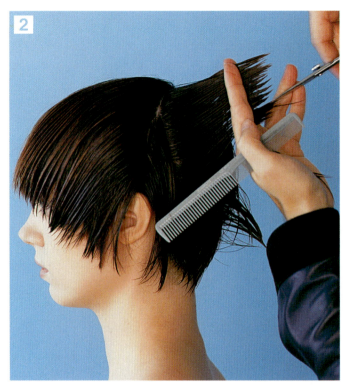

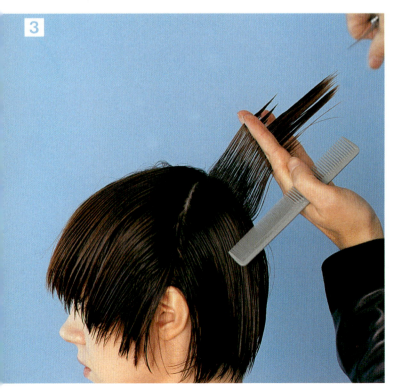

**1** Taking a panel from 2 cm above the occipital bone, cut deep V-sections into the hair, building up a very layered, textured shape.

**2** Continue through the whole back panel.

**3** Continue up to the crown, each V-section is precision cut to maintain a balance as the hair grows out.

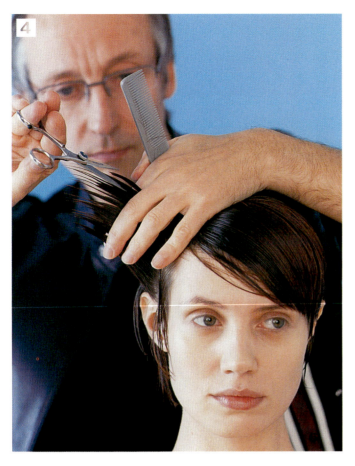

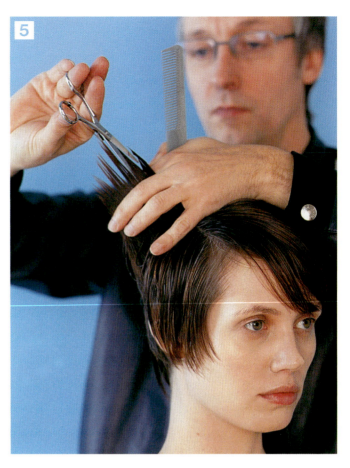

**4** Using the back lengths as your guide, continue into the side panel.

**5** Continue up to the crown building up more length.

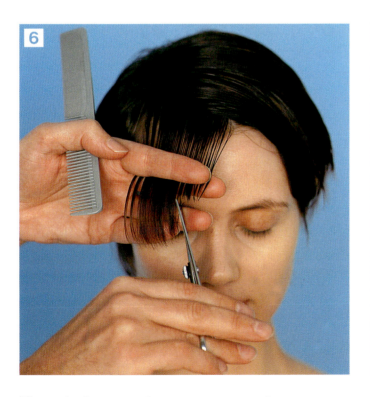

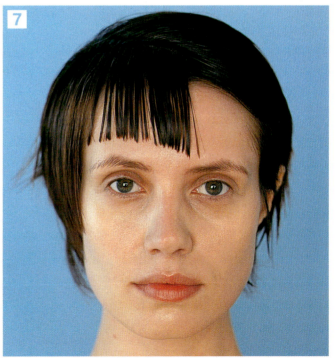

**6** Cut the fringe in a fine point-cutting technique.

**7** Length of fringe established.

# Colouring

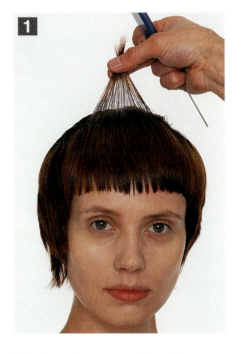

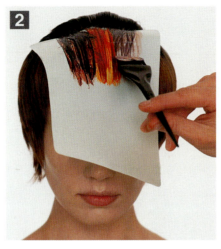

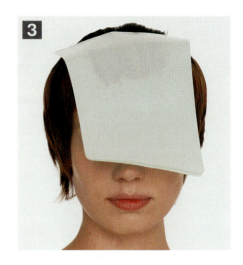

**1** Take a fine section from the crown area. Note that this section is wider then normal.

**2** Place the section on a Creative Colour Wrap and colour using Wella Koleston Perfect 88/43 Vibrant Celtic Copper, Wella Koleston Perfect 55/55 Intense Mahogany, and Wella Koleston Perfect 77/44 Vibrant Fame Red all with 6% Wella Welloxon Perfect Creme Developer.
Note: The edges are overlapped slightly to allow the colours to fuse together.

**3** A Creative Colour Wrap is placed on top of the section to seal.
Note: Creative Colour Wrap follows the head shape allowing a wider section to be taken.

**4** This technique is repeated throughout the top layers.

**5** Wella Koleston Perfect 44/65 Intense Damson Red mixed with 6% Wella Welloxon Perfect Creme Conditioner is applied to the remainder of the hair.

**6** Allow colour to process, then shampoo and condition as normal.

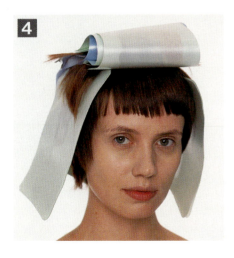

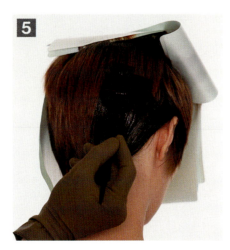

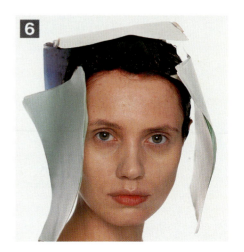

# Finished Look

The hair is dried using Wella SP Styling Spray Lotion and finished using Wella SP Mould & Shine Creme.

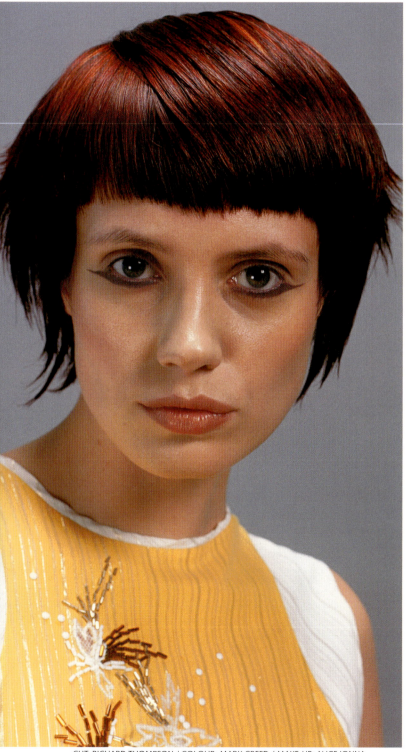

CUT: RICHARD THOMPSON / COLOUR: MARK CREED / MAKE-UP: ALICE IONNA

## Products used

Wella Koleston Perfect:
  88/43 Vibrant Celtic Copper
  55/55 Intense Mahogany
  77/44 Vibrant Flame Red
  44/65 Intense Damson Red

6% Wella Welloxon
Perfect Creme Developer

Wella SP Styling Spray Lotion

Wella SP Mould & Shine Creme

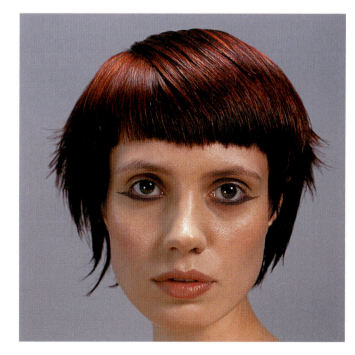

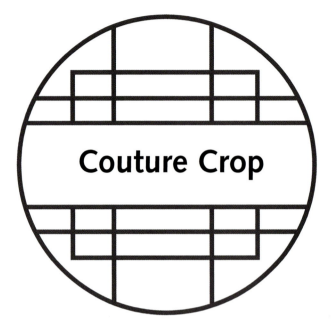

**Couture Crop**

*Extreme point cutting creates space and texture*

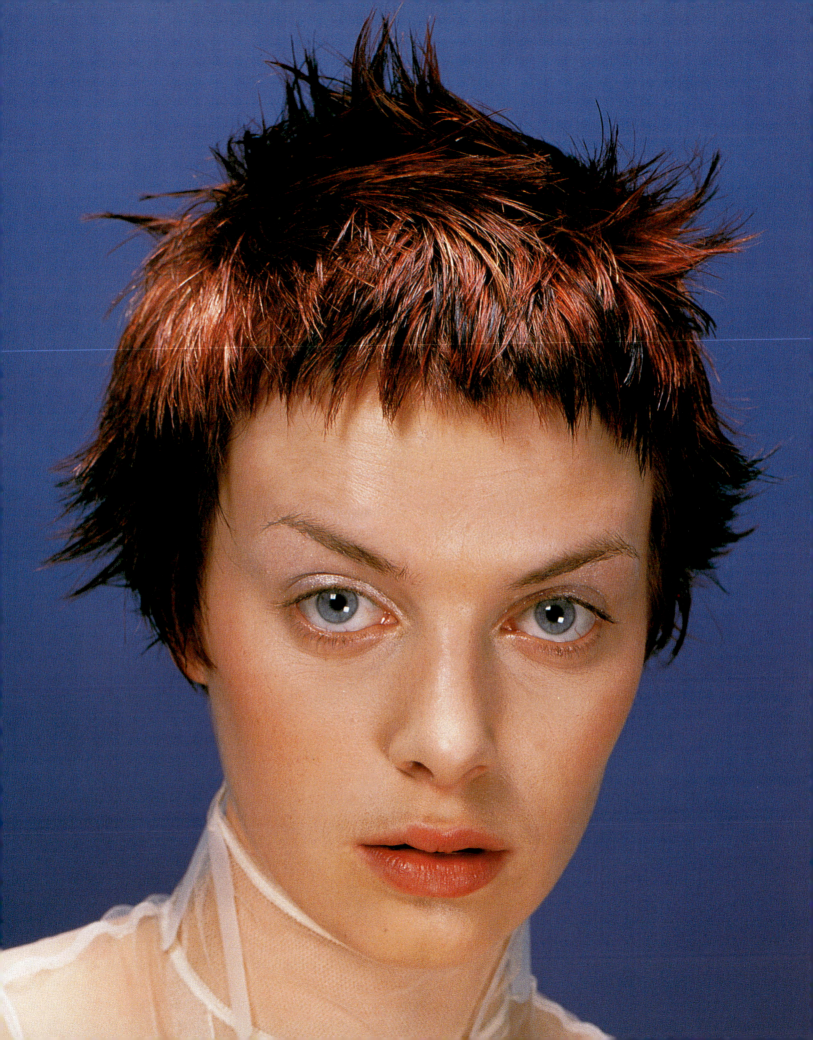

# Cutting

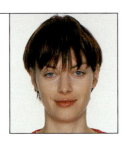

*The model's hair had been cut about four months previously. It had grown out and the model, who likes a strong look, found it uninteresting. After a consultation, it was decided to go for a short chopped cut with strong shadowy colour.*

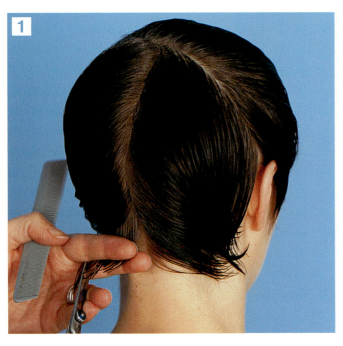

**1** Start the first section in the nape, cut V-sections into the section.

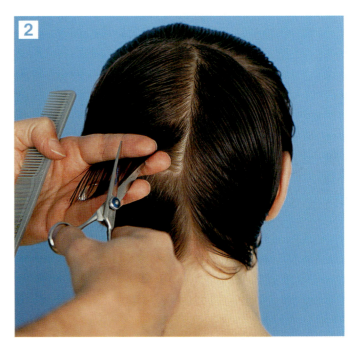

**2** Continue up the back of the head using this technique, always maintaining the internal lengths and external lengths.

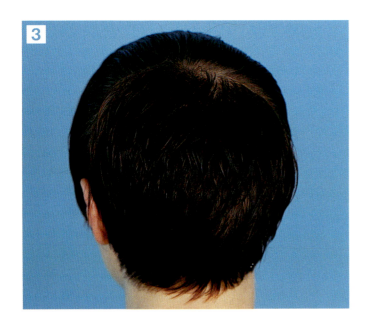

**3** The back is complete.

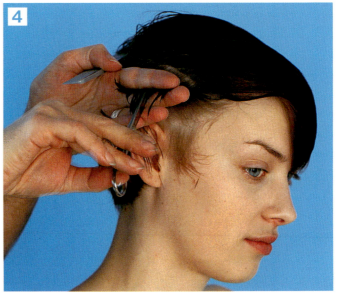

**4** Follow the horizontal sections into the side panel.

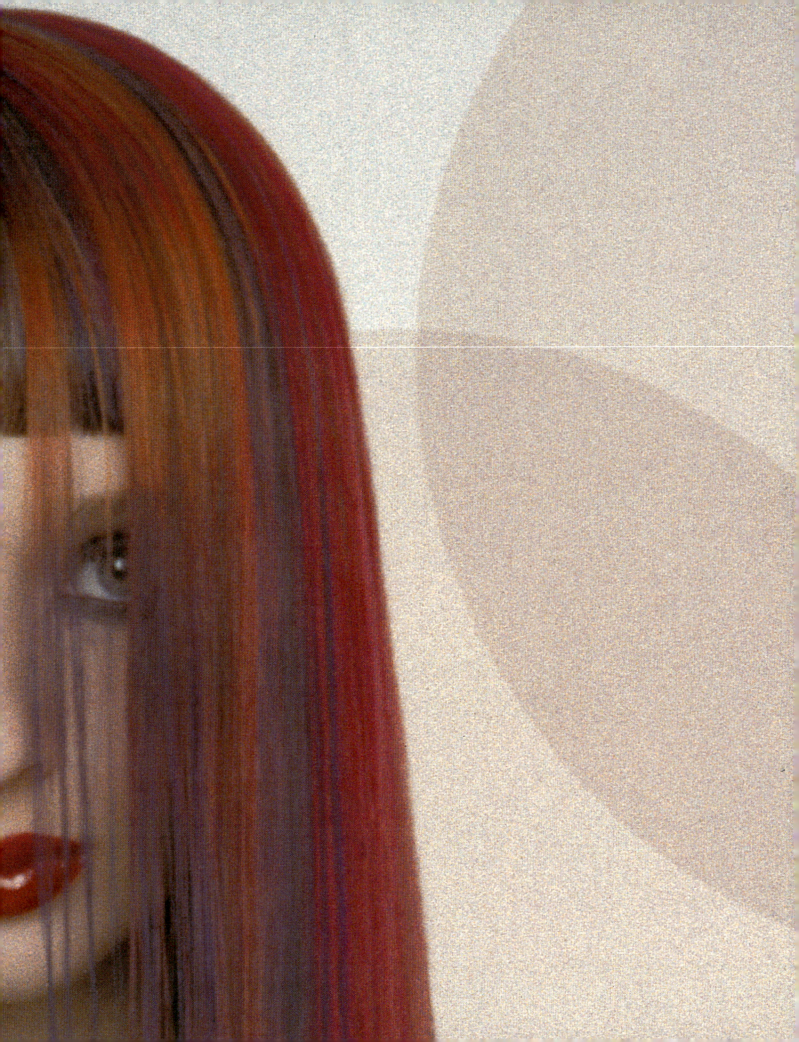

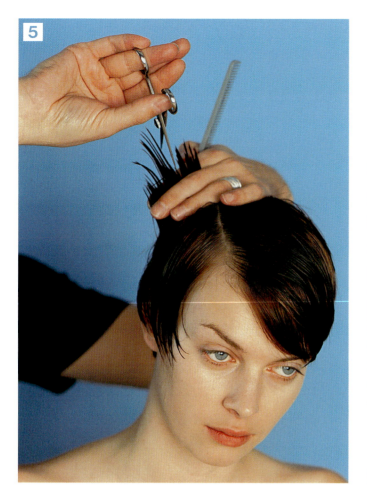

5 Continue to use the V-section technique through the next panels.

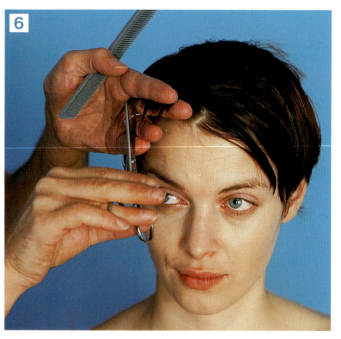

6 Cut the fringe to the desired length.

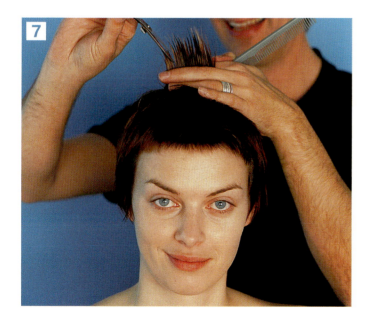

7 Connect the top panels across.

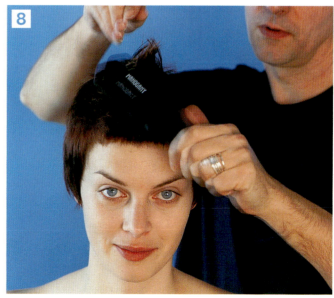

8 Dry the hair using a vent brush to check the balance in the texture.

# Colouring

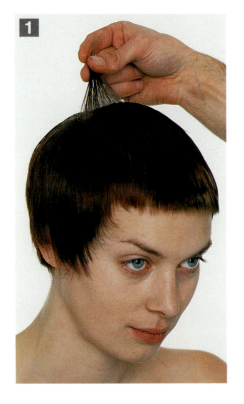

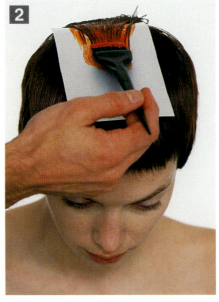

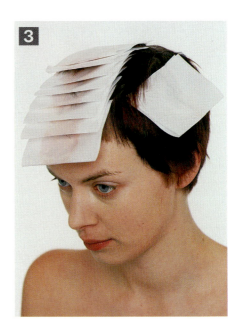

**1** A fine slice is taken from the crown.

**2** A Colour Wrap (cut in half) is placed underneath this section and Wella Koleston Perfect 77/43 Intense Celtic Copper mixed with 6% Welloxon Perfect Creme Developer is applied from roots to ends. A second colour, Wella Koleston Perfect 10/0 Lightest Natural Blonde is then applied directly on top of the previous colour. The Colour Wrap is folded in half to seal the section.

**3** This technique is repeated throughout the top section.

**4** Wella Koleston Perfect 55/46 Vibrant Burgundy Red mixed with 6% Wella Welloxon Perfect Creme Developer is then applied to the rest of the hair.

**5** Finished technique is allowed to process, then shampooed and conditioned as normal.

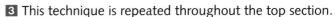

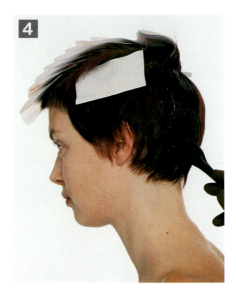

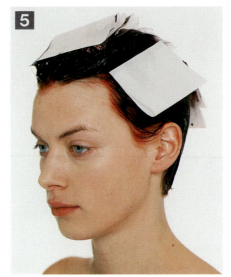

# Finished Look

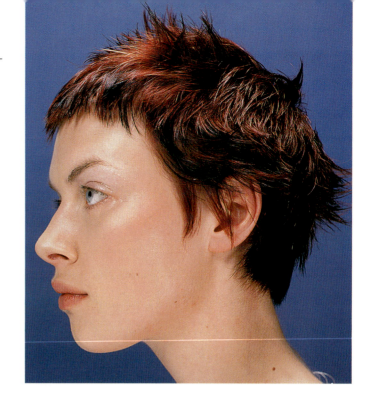

The hair is dried using Wella SP Styling Spray Lotion and finished using Wella SP Mould & Shine Creme.

## Products used

Wella Koleston Perfect:
   77/43 Intense Celtic Copper
   10/0 Lightest Natural Blonde
   55/46 Vibrant Burgundy Red

6% Wella Welloxon
Perfect Creme Developer

9% Wella Welloxon
Perfect Creme Developer

Wella SP Styling Spray Lotion

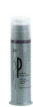

Wella SP Mould & Shine Creme

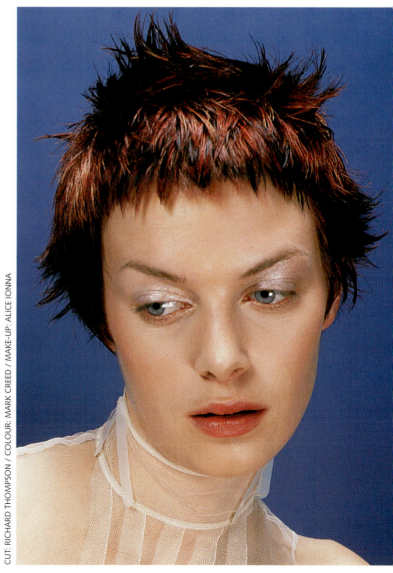

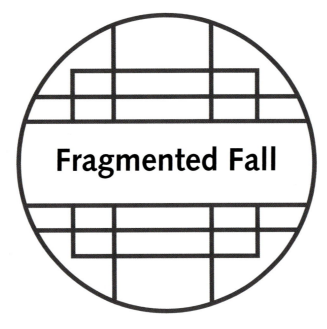

**Fragmented Fall**

*Graduated undercut with freehand tendrils
that trail over sharp outline*

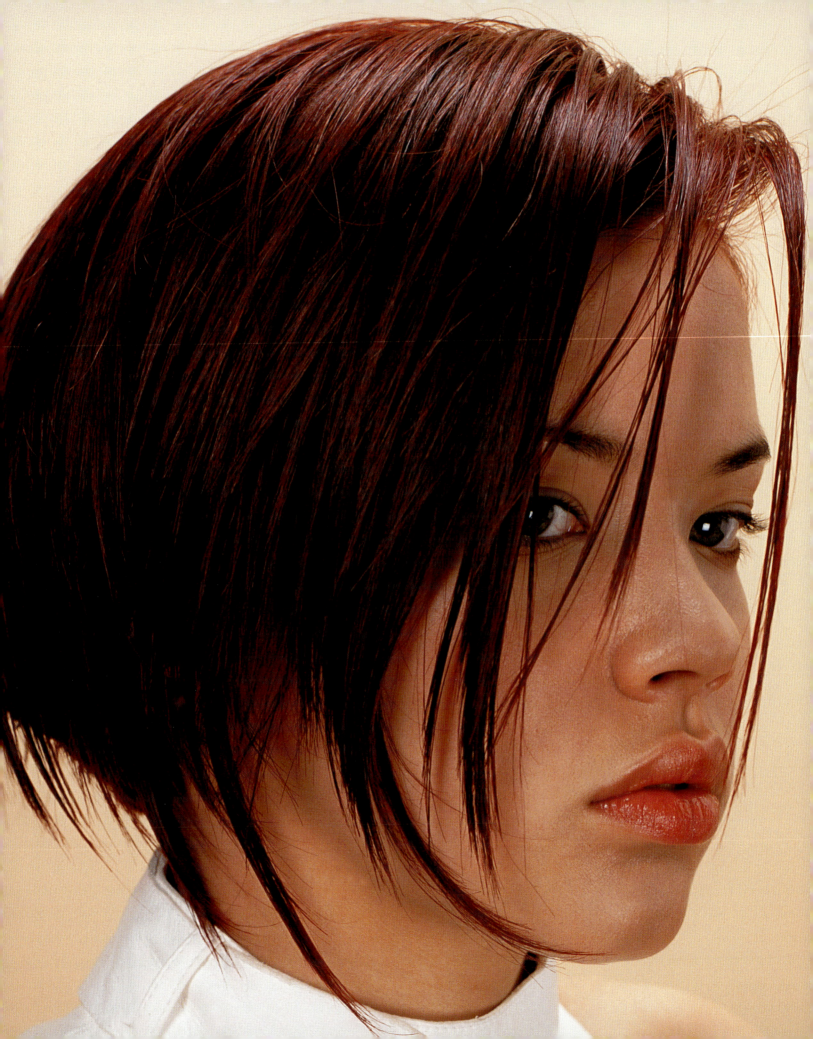

# Colouring

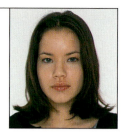

*Fiona's hair was long and straight to her shoulders. After consultation it was decided to go for an undercut shape that could be worn smooth or textured and separated. The colour would be rich reds and enhance the cut shape. The hair was coloured first because the finished look would be difficult to easily section. Her natural colour is 5/0 Light Brown.*

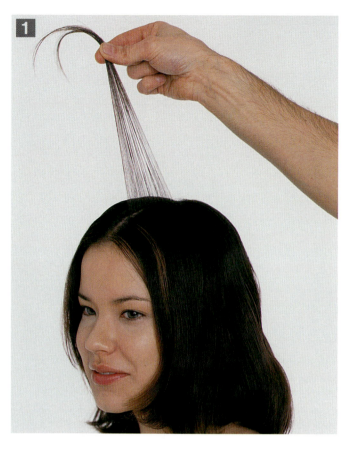

**1** Take a fine slice from the parting.

**2** Place a fine slice on a Colour Wrap and apply Wella Koleston Perfect 6/45 Rich Burgundy Red mixed with 6% Wella Welloxon Creme Developer from roots to ends. Apply two bands of Wella Pure Mixtone 0/45 Red Mix directly on top of this coloured section, at mid-length.

**3** Place a Colour Wrap on top of this section to form a sealed packet.

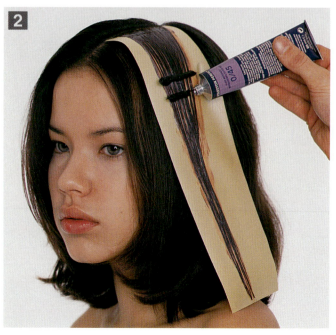

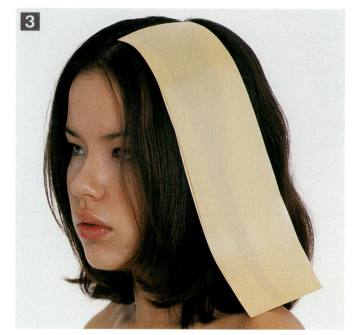

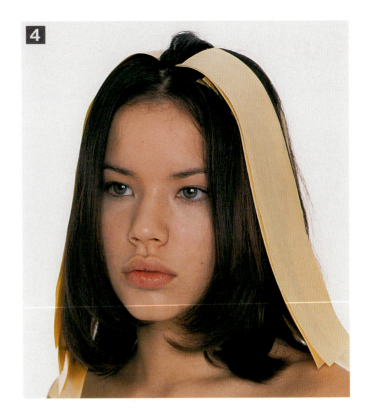

**4** Continue this technique through the top layers.

**5** Wella Koleston Perfect 55/46 Vibrant Burgundy Red mixed with 6% Wella Welloxon Perfect Creme Developer is applied to the rest of the hair.

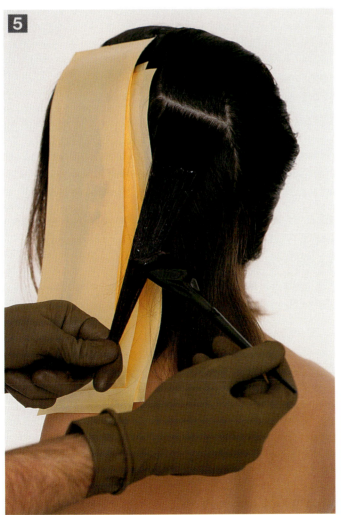

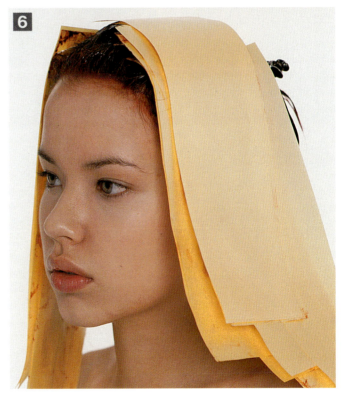

**6** The finished technique is now ready to process. When finished shampoo and condition in the normal way.

The hair is now ready for cutting.

# Cutting

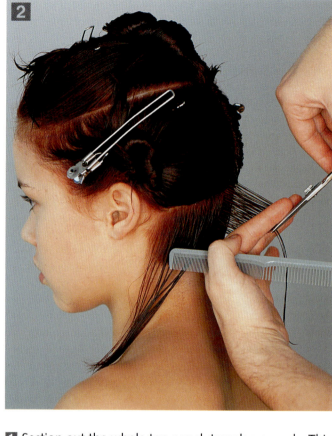

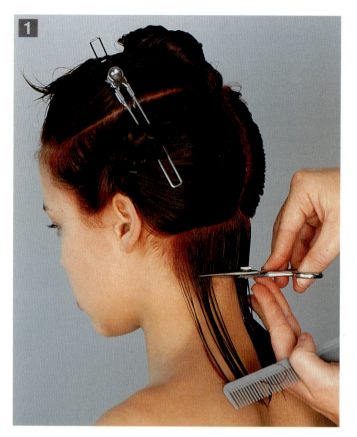

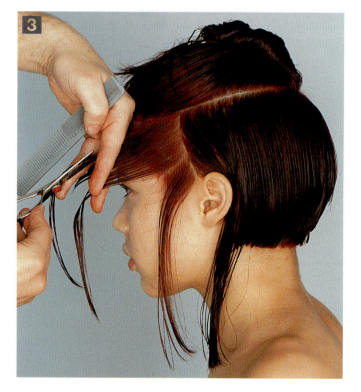

**1** Section out the whole top panel, temple upwards. This hair will be cut dry later. The remaining hair is sectioned as if cutting a square bob, cut your outline length.

**2** Graduate the back, leaving out the section behind the ear.

**3** The graduated back is now complete. Begin parallel to the front hairline cutting an exaggerated angle towards the section you left out behind the ear.

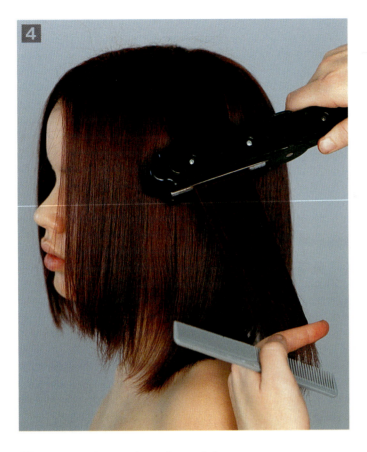

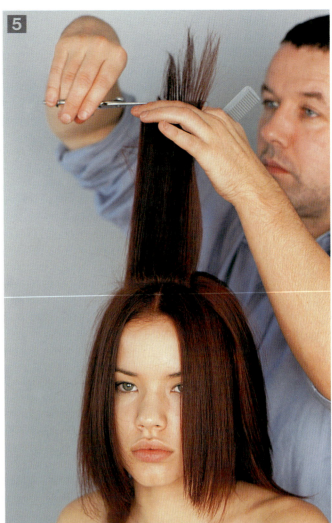

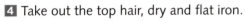 Take out the top hair, dry and flat iron.

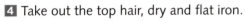 Take a square section across the top and layer to the desired outline length.

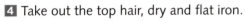 Working around the head, slide cut all edges creating fragmented tendrils.

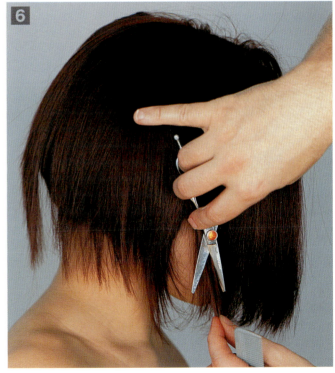

# Finished Look

The hair was dried using Wella SP Styling Spray Lotion and finished with Wella SP Mould & Shine Creme.

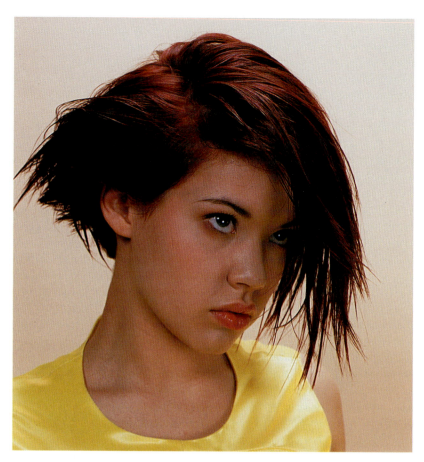

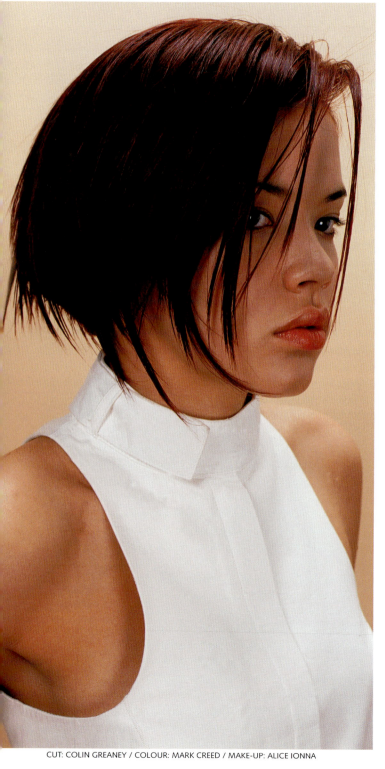

## Products used

Wella Koleston Perfect:
   6/45 Rich Burgundy Red
   55/46 Vibrant Burgundy Red
Wella Pure Mixtone
   0/45 Red Mix

6% Wella Welloxon
Perfect Creme Developer

Wella SP Styling Spray Lotion

Wella SP Mould & Shine Creme

CUT: COLIN GREANEY / COLOUR: MARK CREED / MAKE-UP: ALICE IONNA

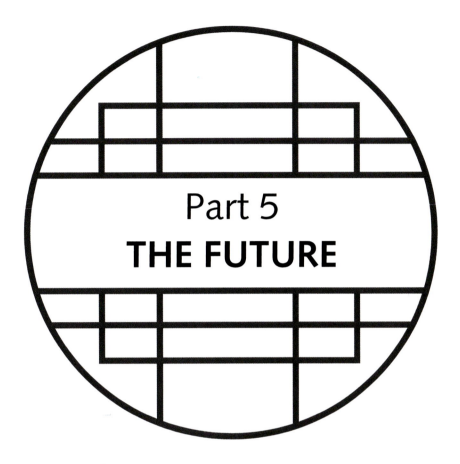

# Part 5
# THE FUTURE

*Where does it start, where does it finish?*

*The hidden techniques of cut and colour.*

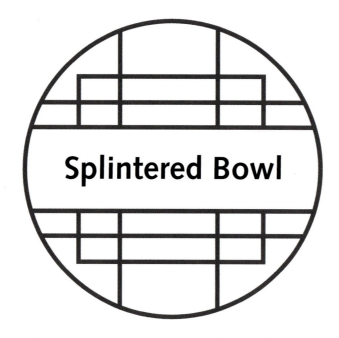

**Splintered Bowl**

*A sharp, asymmetric bowl outline interjected with disconnected tails*

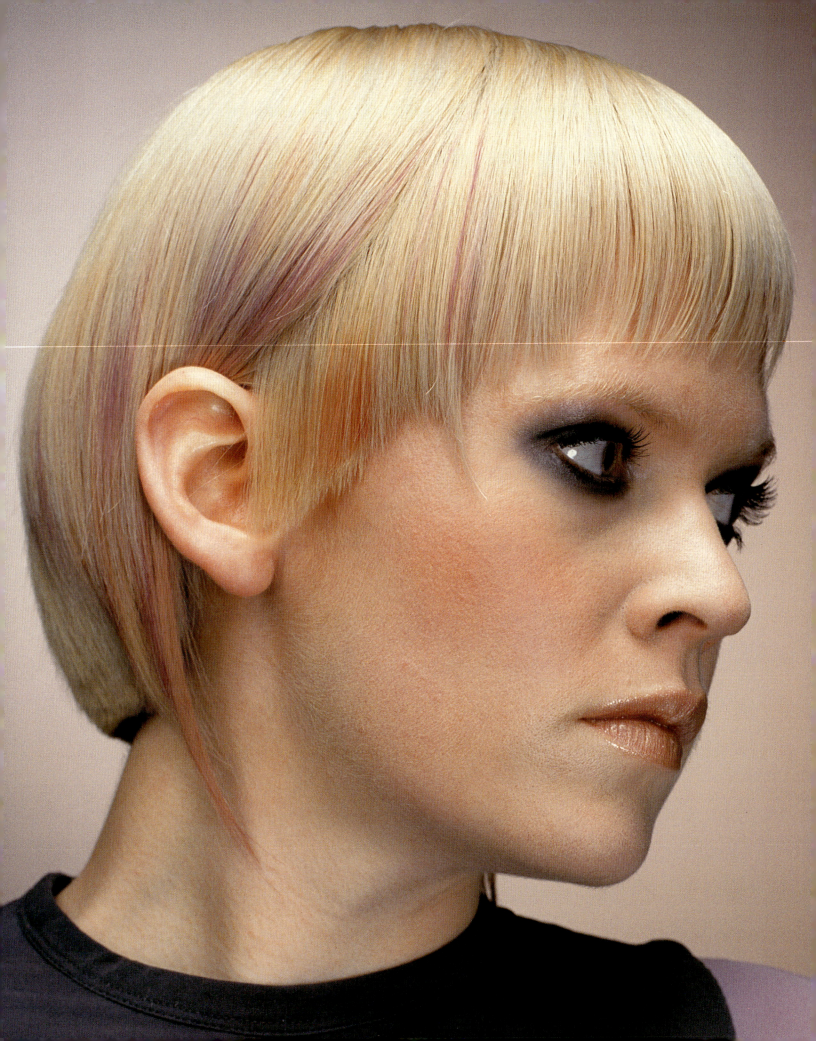

# Cutting

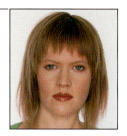

*Our model's hair was in a grown-out bob shape. She wanted to be blonde and have a radical look.*

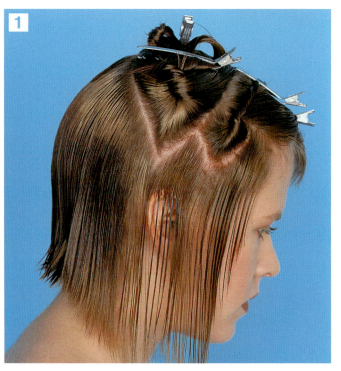

**1** Section out two triangular panels.

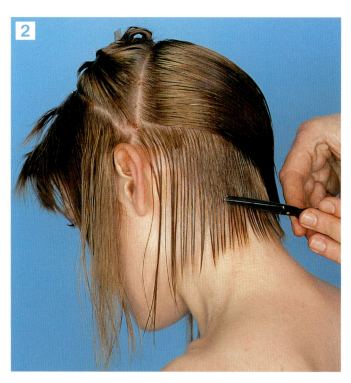

**2** Cut a base line up towards the back of the ear.

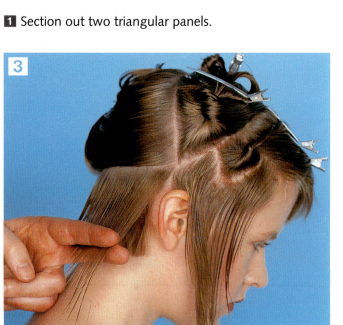

**3** Create horizontal graduation by lifting hair to a finger width from the neck.

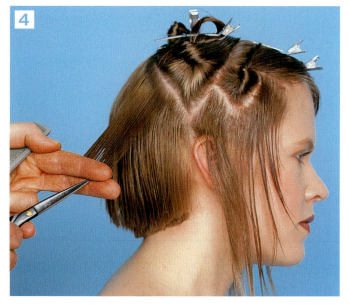

**4** Continue up to the crown and back of the triangular panel. Point cut last section to soften edge.

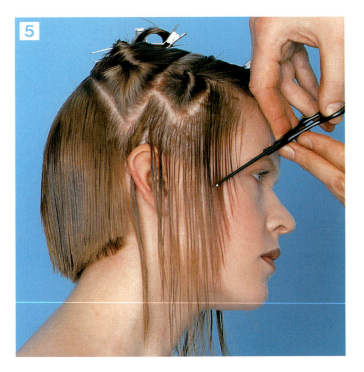

5 Cut a line from the temple to meet nape line.

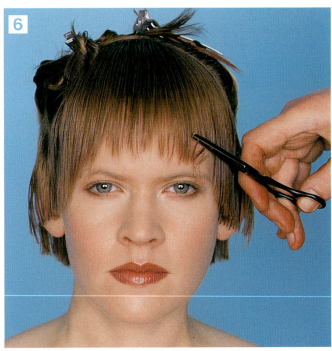

6 Cut a high line on the right-hand side of the fringe, the left side of the fringe will be stepped from this line.

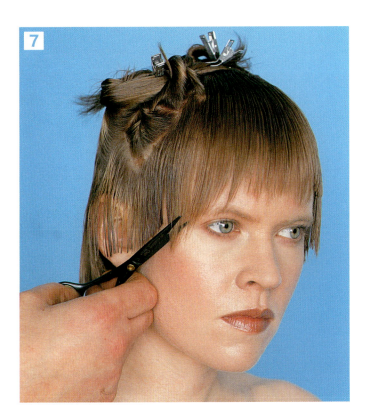

7 Cut opposite side.

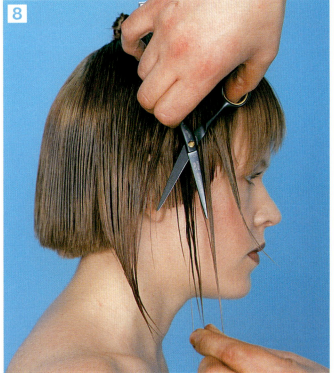

8 Take down triangular panels and visually slice into the outline.
Note: There is no clear distinction between right and wrong for the final look. Visually, you are creating a balance that fits with the strong cut outline

# Colouring

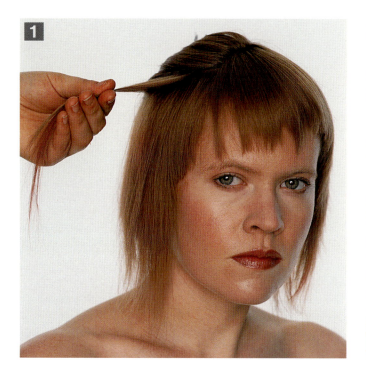

**1** Take a fine slice from the underneath layers of hair.

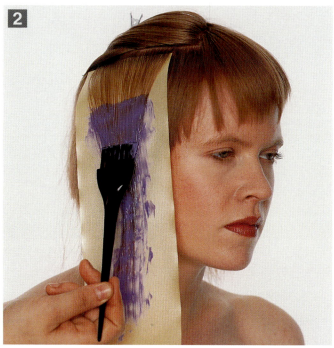

**2** Place the hair on a Colour Wrap and apply Wella Koleston Perfect 6/6 Sherry Brown mixed with 6% Wella Welloxon Perfect Creme Developer to lengths and ends.

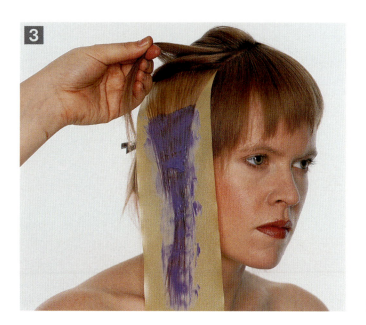

**3** Take a 2 cm section and clip out to the side, then take another fine slice above this.

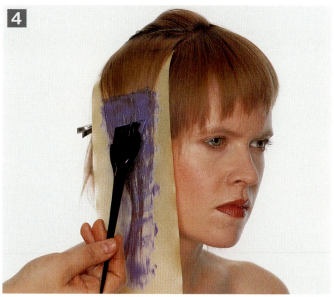

**4** Lay this fine slice directly on top of the previously coloured slice and apply Wella Koleston Perfect 8/4 Sunset Red to the mid-lengths and ends.

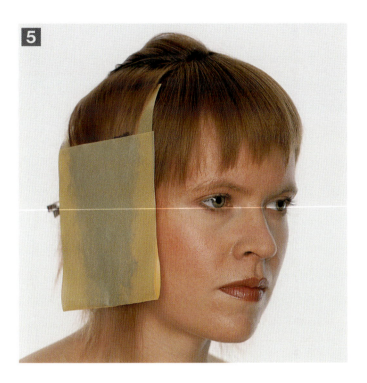

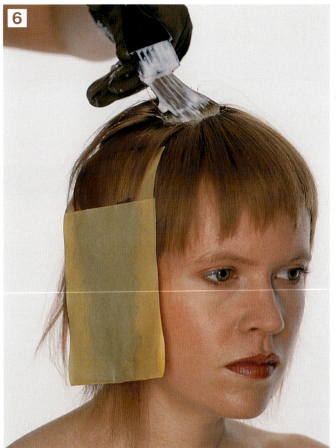

**5** Fold the Colour Wrap to seal sections. Repeat this on the other side of the head.

**6** Apply a high lift clear blonde to the rest of the hair using Wella Koleston Perfect 12/16 Special Soft Ash mixed with 12% Wella Welloxon Perfect Creme Developer.

**7** The finished technique is now ready to process. When finished, shampoo and condition as normal.

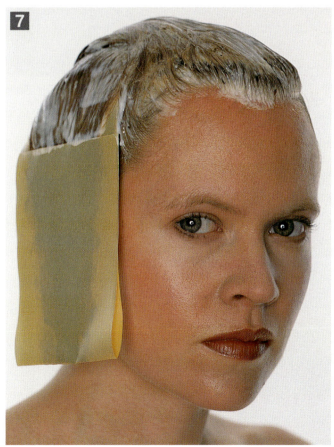

# Finished Look

The hair is finished with Mahogany Mini Flatteners and Wella SP Ends Express is applied for shine.

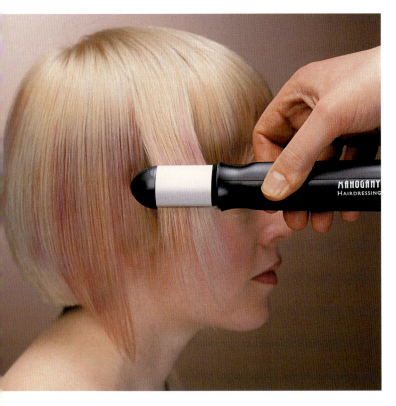

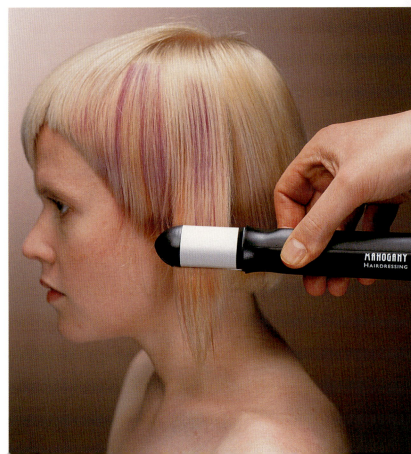

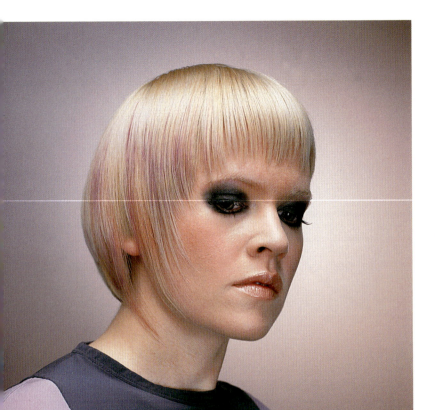

## Products used

Wella Koleston Perfect:
6/6 Sherry Brown
12/16 Special Soft Ash

6% Wella Welloxon
Perfect Creme Developer

12% Wella Welloxon
Perfect Creme Developer

Wella SP Ends Express

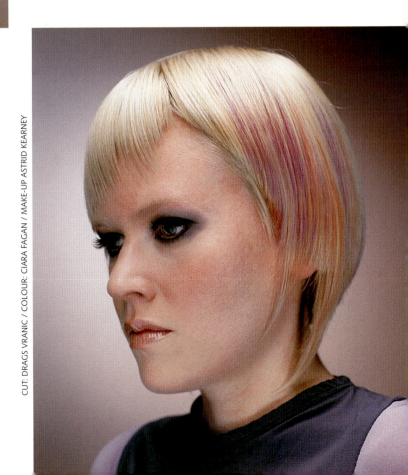

CUT: DRAGS VRANIC / COLOUR: CIARA FAGAN / MAKE-UP ASTRID KEARNEY

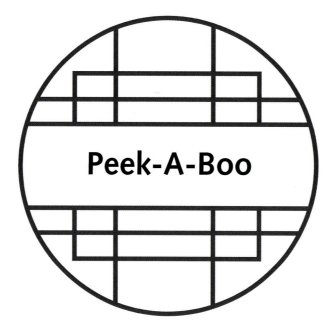

**Peek-A-Boo**

*Graphic outline with ultimate disconnection
and a peek-a-boo fringe*

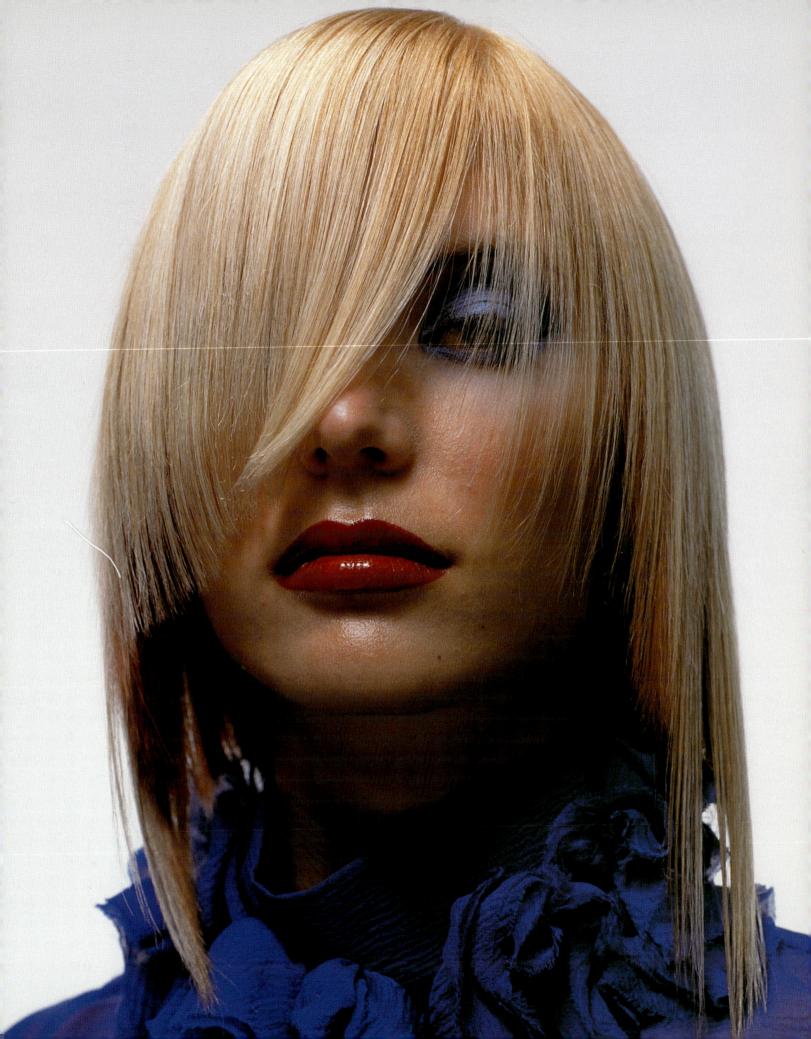

# Cutting

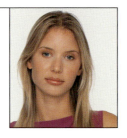

*Our model's hair is long and highlighted.
She wants a more dramatic cut and colour.*

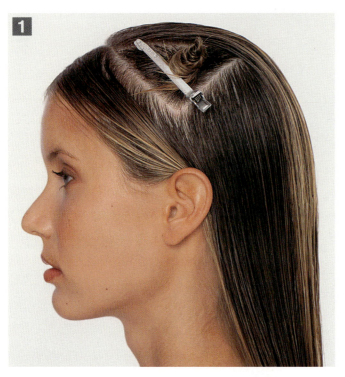

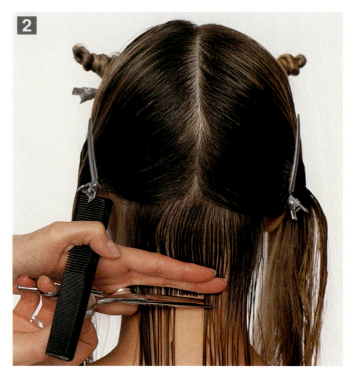

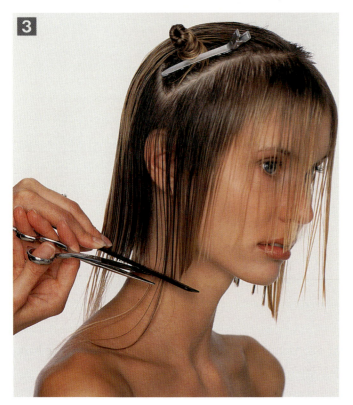

**1** Section a triangle out on either side approximately 2 cm above the top of the ear and 2 cm from the central parting.

**2** Establish a square outline length.

**3** Continue the line into the side panel.

Repeat on opposite side.

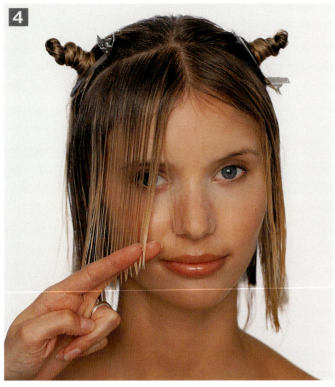

**4** Cut an angle upwards in line with the bottom of the nose.

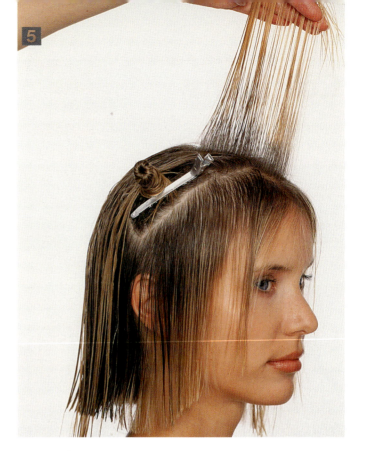

**5** Layer the top sections using the shortest point at the front as your guide.

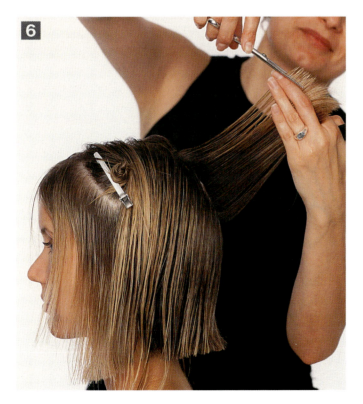

**6** Holding the section parallel to the head shape, layer off the back corner. Now let down the triangular panels and dry the hair.

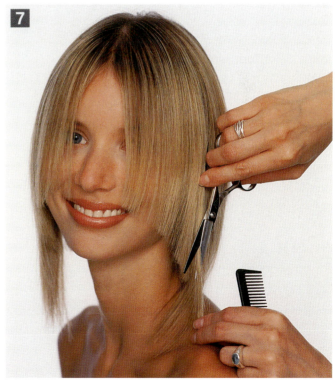

**7** Slide cut the triangular panels into the rest of the hair creating a visual balance.

# Colouring

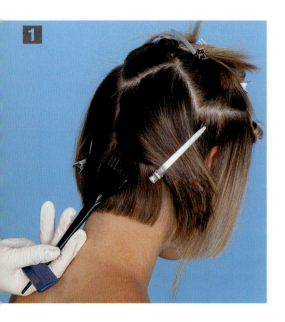

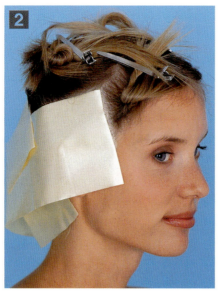

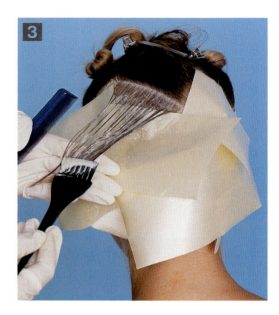

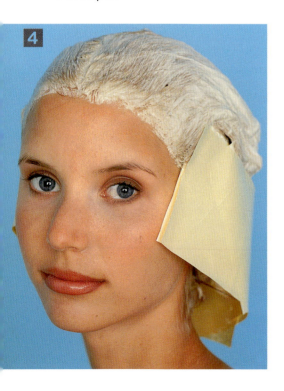

**1** Take a zig-zag section around the head and clip the top layers out of the way. Colour the underneath sections using Wella Color Touch Intensive Red 77/45 mixed with Wella Color Touch Intensive Lotion Developer.

**2** Cover the underneath coloured sections with Colour Wraps for protection.

**3** Colour the remaining top hair with Wella Koleston Perfect 12/16 Special Soft Ash mixed with 12% Wella Welloxon Perfect Creme Developer.

**4** The finished technique is now ready to process. When finished shampoo and condition as normal.

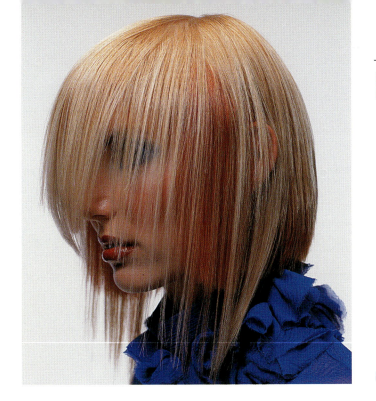

# Finished Look

Hair is dried with Wella Controlling Spray.

## Products used

Wella Color Touch Intensive
Red 77/45

Wella Color Touch Intensive
Creme Lotion

Wella Koleston Perfect:
12/16 Special Soft Ash

12% Wella Welloxon
Perfect Creme Developer

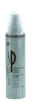

Wella SP Controlling Spray

CUT: MAHOGANY CREATIVE TEAM / COLOUR: KEERA FAGAN / MAKE-UP: ASTRID KEARNEY

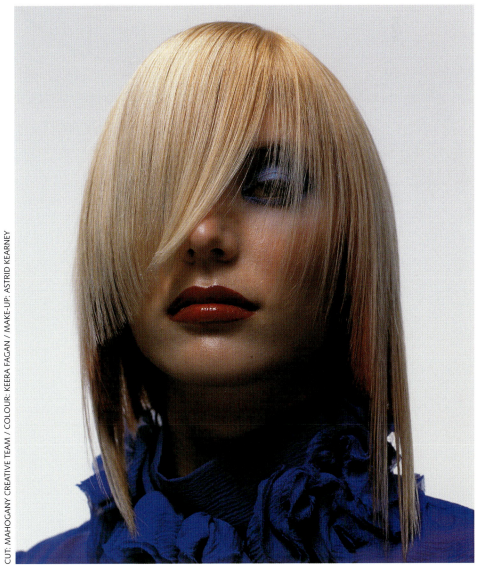

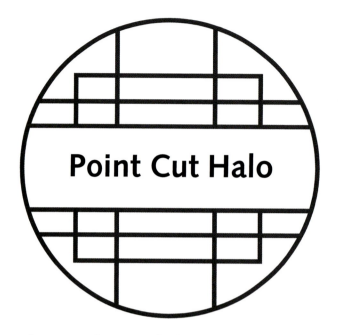

**Point Cut Halo**

Texturing the outline of this undercut bowl shape
enables it to be worn flicked or smooth

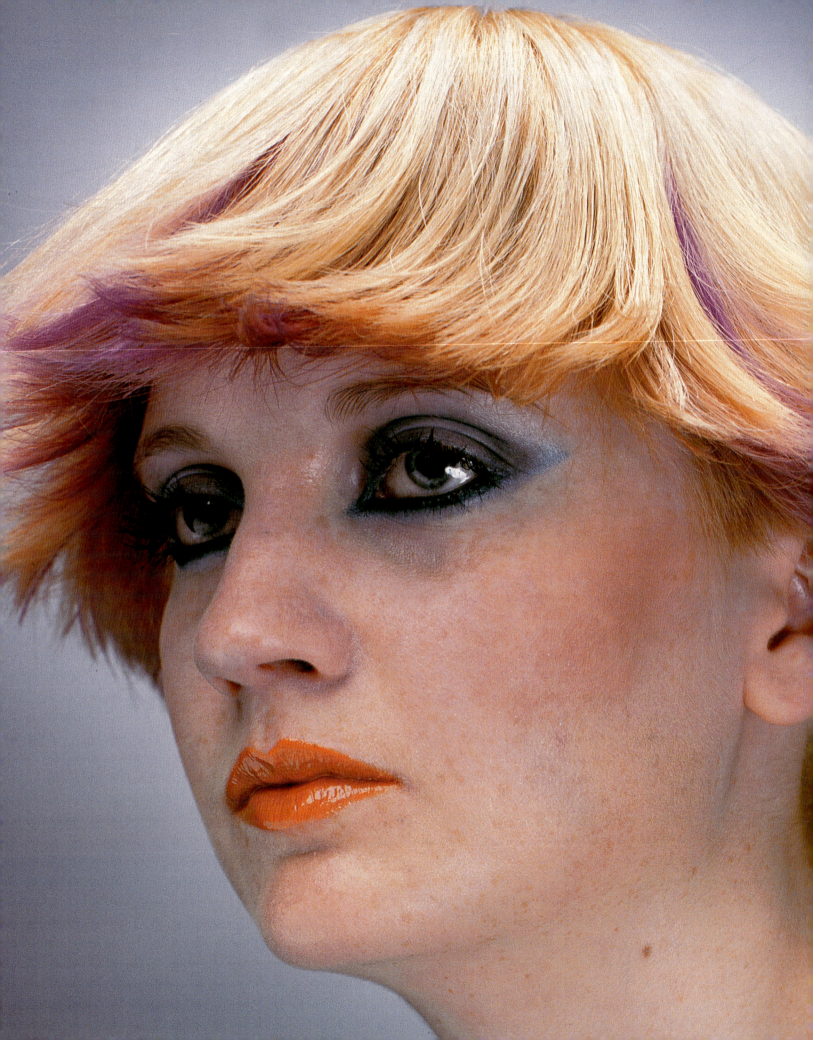

# Colouring

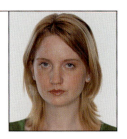

*Our model's hair was grown out and shapeless. She wants to be blonder and have a shorter but versatile cut.*

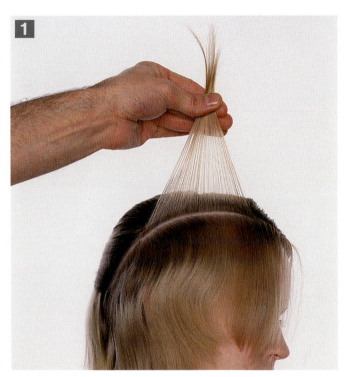

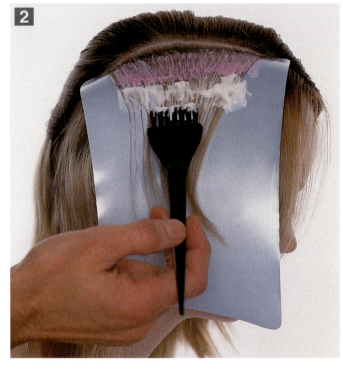

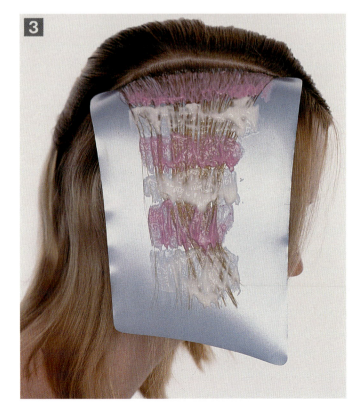

**1** Take a slice from a parting approximately 2 cm under natural parting.

**2** Place a Creative Colour Wrap under slice. Alternate each colour in bands of approximately 2 cm using Wella Koleston Perfect 55/46 Vibrant Burgundy Red and Wella 10/0 Lightest Blonde both mixed with 6% Wella Welloxon Perfect Creme Developer.

**3** Finished application to first slice.

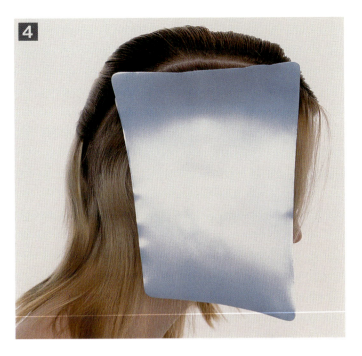

**4** Cover with a second Creative Colour Wrap.

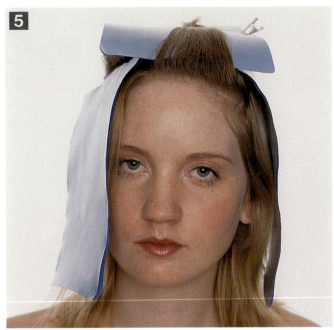

**5** Continue this technique in a circular shape around the head 2 cm below natural parting, 2 cm below crown and 1 cm from front hairline.

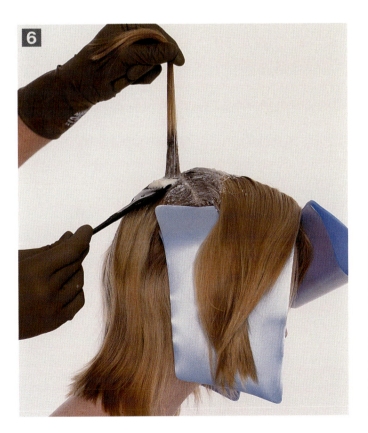

**6** Apply Wella Koleston Perfect 12/1 Special Ash Blonde and 12% Wella Welloxon Perfect Creme Developer.

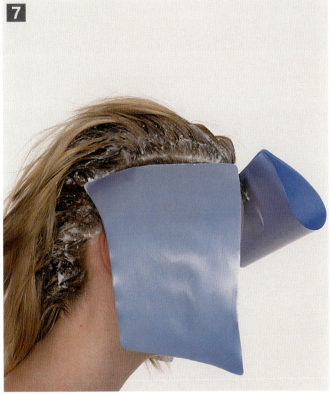

**7** Allow to process, then shampoo and condition as normal.
Note: Creative Colour Wraps fit the shape of the head allowing for longer slices to be taken.

# Cutting

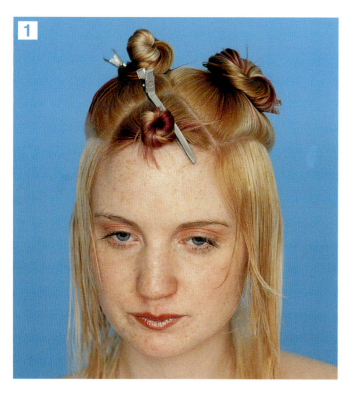

**1** Section away top hair in panels as shown.

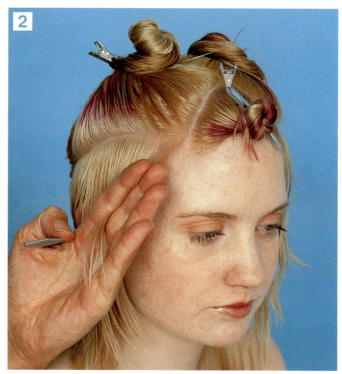

**2** Undercut the underneath hair to finger width.

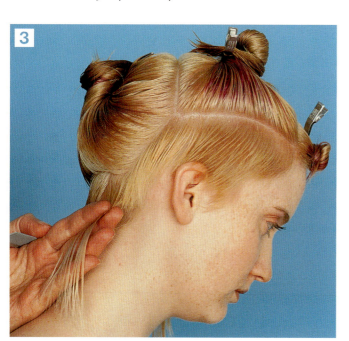

**3** Continue into nape.

**4** Finished undercut.

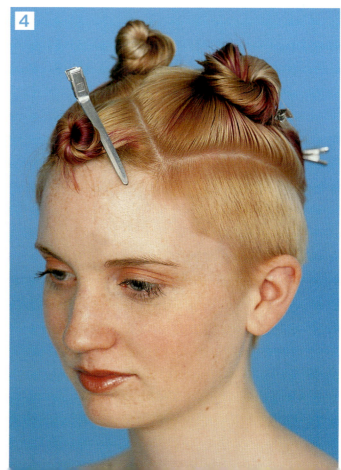

132

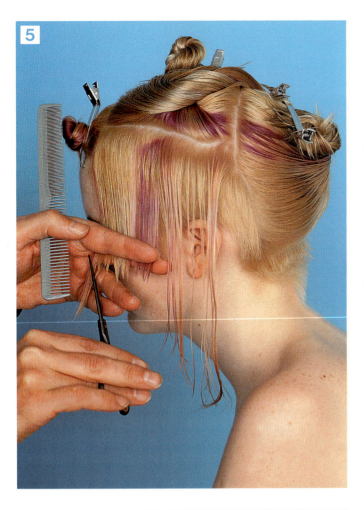

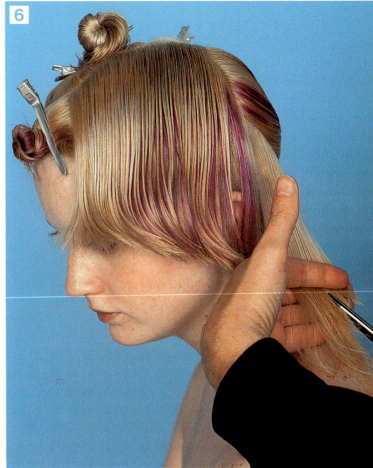

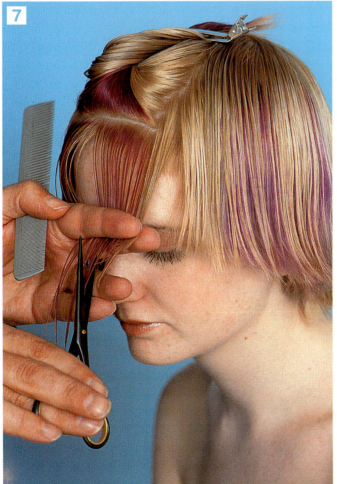

**5** Begin a new line cutting V-sections into the desired lengths to create a diffused outline.

**6** Continue on opposite side and into the nape, creating a halo shaped outline.

**7** Continue into fringe creating the same texture, cutting to a length that can be worn straight or flicked.

# Finished Look

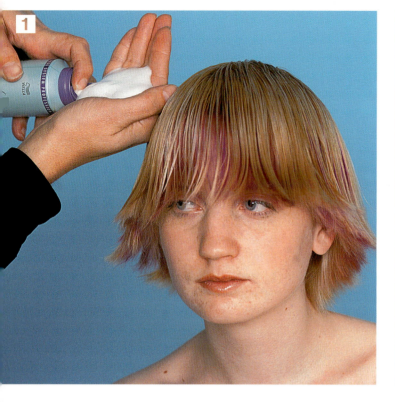

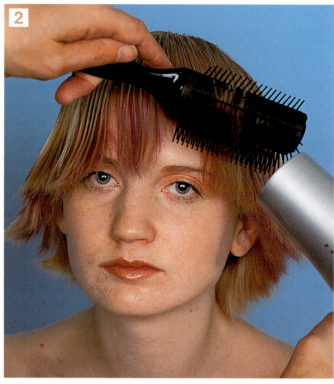

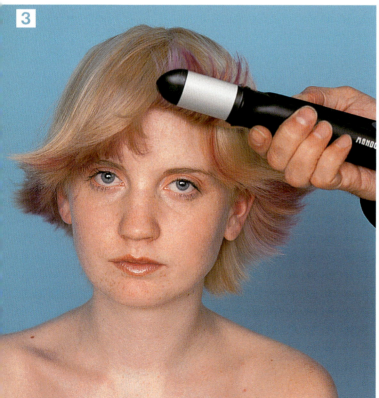

**1** Apply Wella SP Texturising Mousse before drying.

**2** Dry, tipping the ends out and back.

**3** Use Mahogany Mini Flatteners to achieve a silk slick finish.

Note: If you pull straight downwards they will flatten hair. If you lift up they will create a straight modern flick.

## Products used

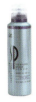

Wella Koleston Perfect:
   55/46 Vibrant Burgundy Red
   10/0 Lightest Blonde
   12/1 Special Ash Blonde

6% Wella Welloxon
Perfect Creme Developer

12% Wella Welloxon
Perfect Creme Developer

Wella SP Texturising Mousse

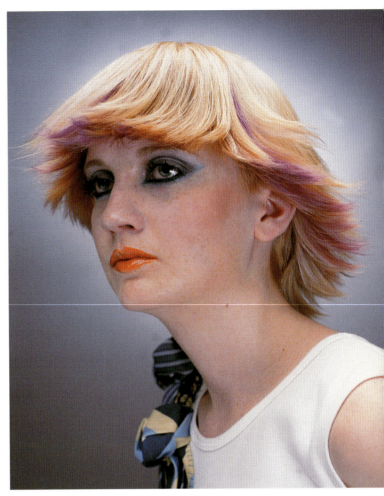

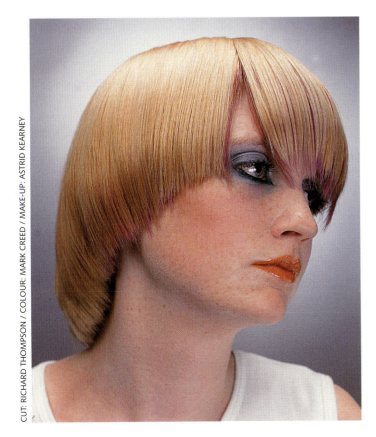

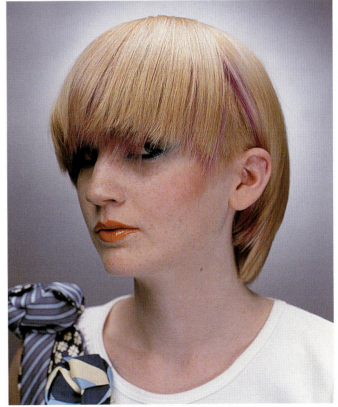

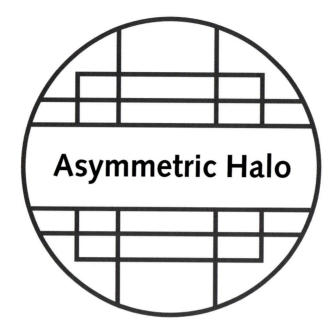

**Asymmetric Halo**

*Working with multiple graphic lines
creates the ultimate asymmetric silhouette*

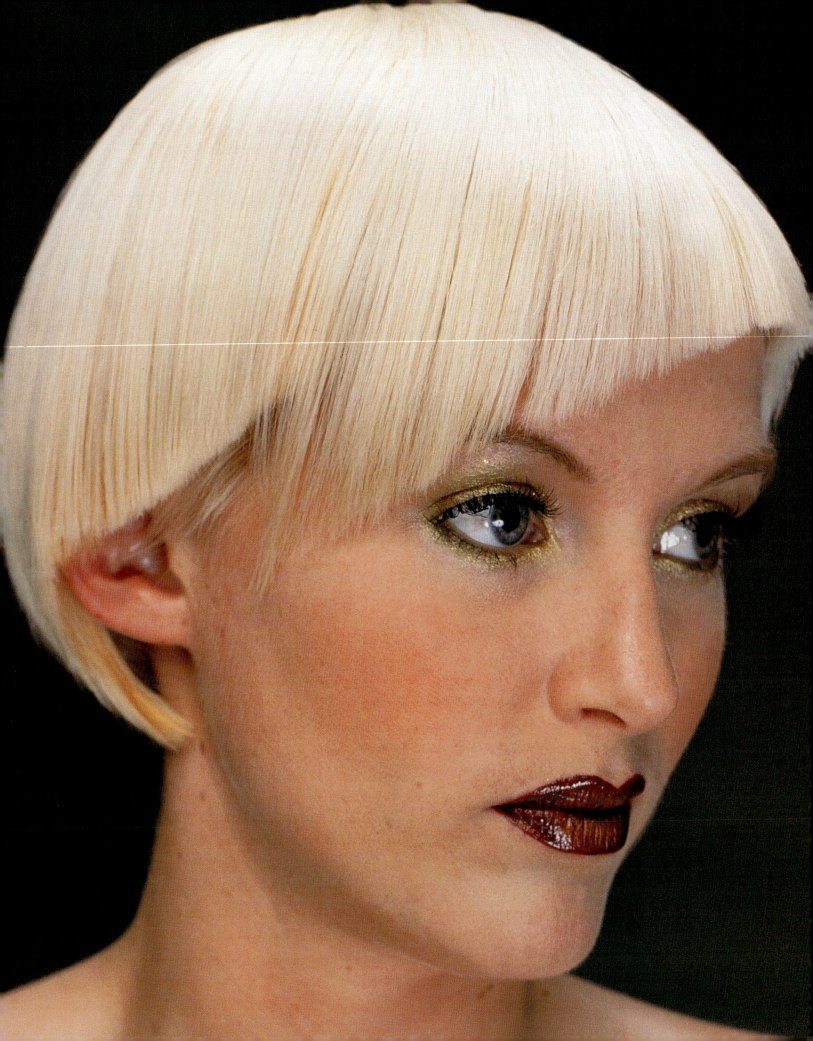

# Colouring

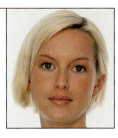

*Our model's hair is cut into a short bob shape. She stipulated that she wanted a totally dramatic shape and colour.*

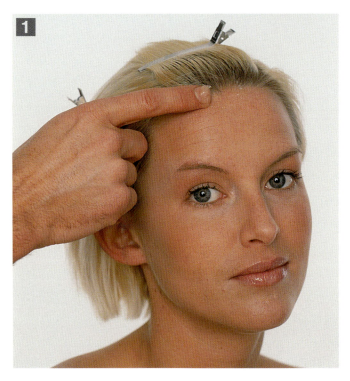

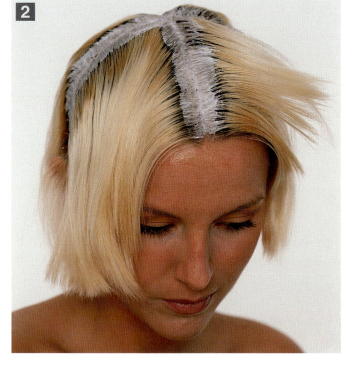

1 Apply skin guard around hairline to protect the skin from the bleach.

2 Section hair into four panels and taking fine sections in each panel carefully apply bleach to regrowth only using Wella Blondor Special and 6% Wella Welloxon Perfect Creme Developer.

3 Use cotton wool to separate the sections. This prevents overlay of bleach on hair lengths.

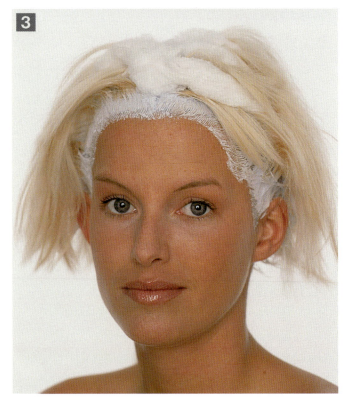

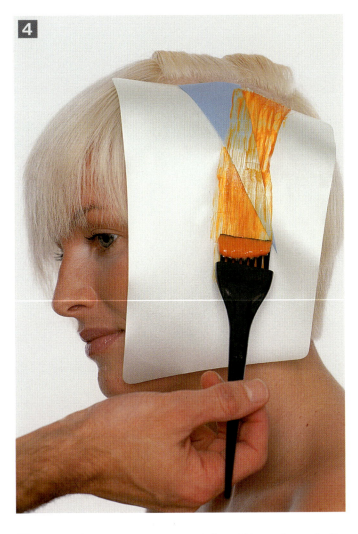

**4** Place a slice onto a Creative Colour Wrap. Cover half the slice with a long triangular piece of Colour Wrap, and apply Wella Koleston Perfect 8/73 Golden Sand and 6% Wella Welloxon Perfect Creme Developer to the rest of the hair.

**5** Take three slices on each side. The effect created will be diffused saffron shades. The stencil of the long cover triangle masks areas of your choice for the desired effect.

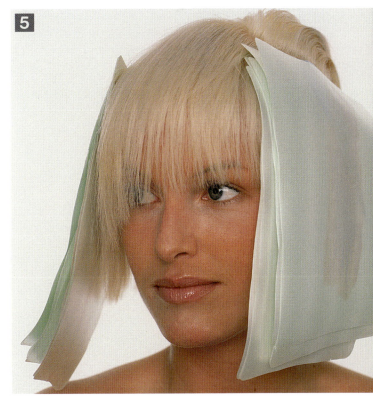

# Cutting

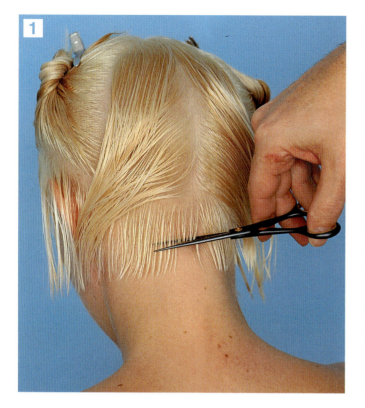

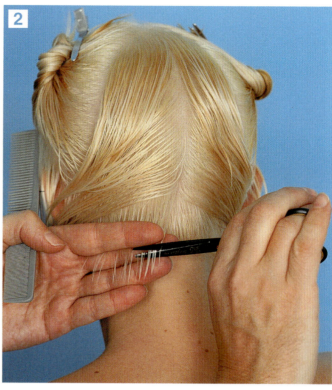

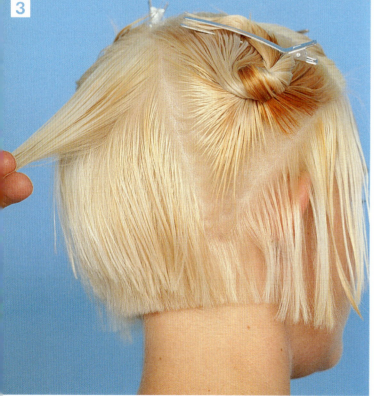

**1** Cut a square base line.

**2** Lift following sections to create horizontal graduation.

**3** Continue up, maintaining the horizontal graduation to the same degree.

Note: When using the horizontal graduation technique make sure the head stays in the same position, a change of position will result in an uneven angle of graduation.

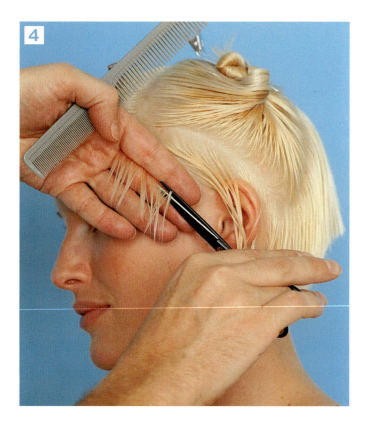

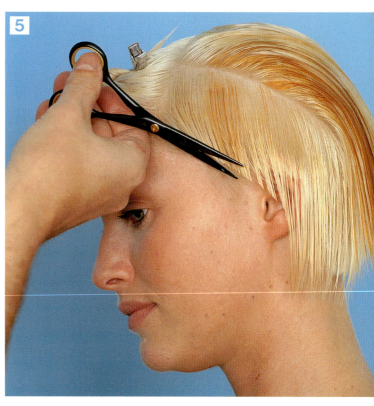

**4** Cut a line lifting hair between the fingers from temple hair to mid-ear.

**5** Using the line at the top of the graduation created from the previous section cut a freehand line with no graduation from the temple to the length behind the ear.

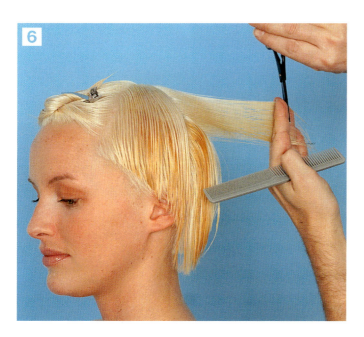

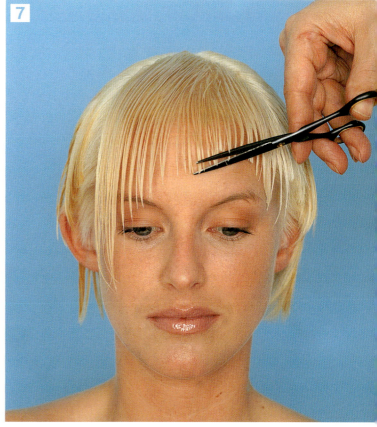

**6** Check the sides into the back using the last section of the back as your guide.

**7** Cut an asymmetric halo-shaped fringe. Check sides of the fringe with the temple to create a stepped effect at the side of the fringe and temples.

# Finished Look

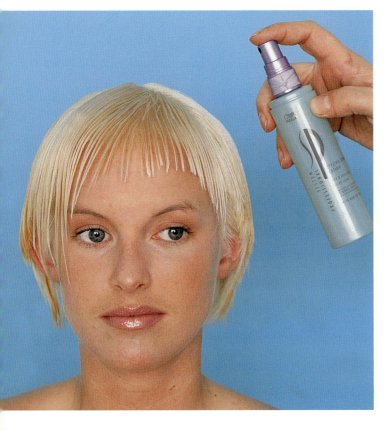

Spray Wella SP Styling Spray Lotion onto hair before drying.

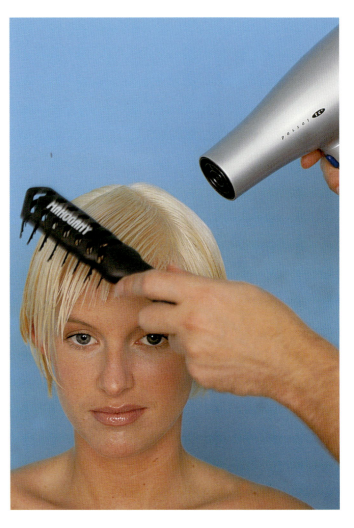

Dry using a Mahogany Vent Brush. Finish for shine with Wella SP Ends Express.

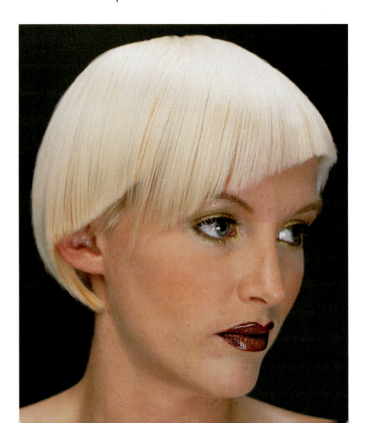

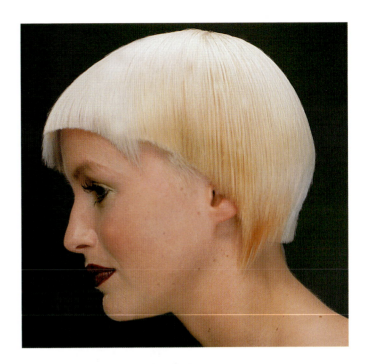

## Products used

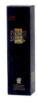

Wella Blondor Special Creme

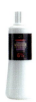

6% Wella Welloxon
Perfect Creme Developer

Wella Koleston Perfect:
8/73 Golden Sand

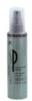

Wella SP Styling Spray Lotion

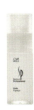

Wella SP Ends Express

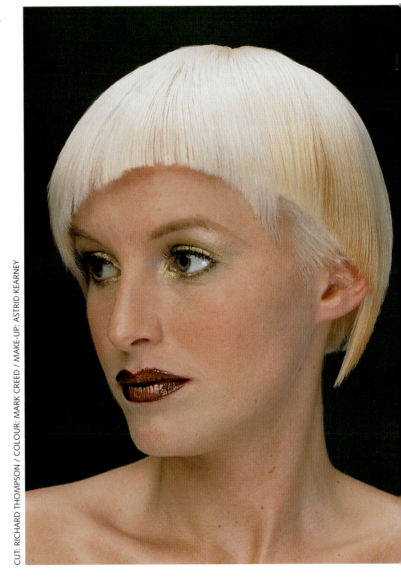

CUT: RICHARD THOMPSON / COLOUR: MARK CREED / MAKE-UP: ASTRID KEARNEY

143

# Glossary

**BANDING**

When a band of colour is placed on the head to appear as a vertical stripe.

**BRUSHES**

Ceramic:
Ceramic pins allow for tangle-free, sleek brushing. The base minimises static.

Vent: A hollow brush head with a wide-spaced pin formation separated by chevron vents, increases the air flow to the hair, providing movement and root lift.

**COLOUR/PERM TECHNICIAN**

A hairdressing specialist. An expert who has full knowledge, technical and artistic ability and is responsible for the colour/perm department.

**COLOUR WRAP**

A Mahogany product, made from a lightweight thermal expanded polypropolene, which is used for colouring hair.
Note: gloves are not worn when colouring on Colour Wraps. Gloves are worn when applying colour direct to hair.

**CREATIVE COLOUR WRAP**

A unique shaped Colour Wrap. It has wide-shaped edges that fit the shape of the head.

**CONSULTATION**

Initial period with client to listen, advise, direct and explain styling, colouring, perming and conditioning.

**DEEP DIVISION**

A deep triangular section of hair that only visually checks with other sections.

**GRADUATION**

When the under hair is shorter than the top lengths, i.e. cut at less than a 90 degree angle to the side or back of the head.

**HIGHLIGHTING**

Weaving in of colour that is then placed either in Colour Wraps or foil. The colour is lifted lighter than the base colour.

**LAYERING**

When all the hair is cut to the same length at 90 degrees to the head shape. The internal lengths may be shorter than the external lengths, i.e. cut at more than 90 degrees to the sides or back.

**LOWLIGHTING**

Weaving in of colour that is then placed either in Colour Wraps or foil. The colour added is richer or deeper than the base colour.

**MINI FLATTENERS**

Ultra sleek mini irons used to straighten and flatten hair. Ideal for close hair-line work.

**ONE LENGTH**

When the outline is one line. All the hair following from a parting to the outside length forms one line

**OVER DIRECT**

To hold subsequent sections to the first section so that they are no longer at 90 degrees to the head, thereby building more length through these sections. This can be done forwards or backwards.

**OVERLAY CUTTING**

To cut by sliding your scissors over the hair in a tapering movement rather than cutting a sharp blunt edge.

**PADDLE BRUSH**

Flat-backed hairbrush with a 5" x 4" bristle area, ideal for smoothing hair and creating a flat shiny finish.

## PANEL

A large section of the head, e.g. ear to ear below the occipital bone.

## POINT CUTTING

To serrate the ends of the hair by cutting fine, sharp V-sections

## ROUNDED GRADUATION

To work the lengths around the shape of the head, not forming any square corners.

## SECTION

A width of hair taken from a panel, approximately 1cm wide.

## SEGMENTING

When a specific shape of colour – elliptical or triangular – is placed into the hair.

## SLICING

When you colour the whole section taken before you weave for highlights or lowlights.

## SLIDE CUTTING

To allow the scissor blades to cut into the hair by sliding down the lengths of the hair.

## SQUARE GRADUATION

To maintain a square line held at just below 90 degrees to the head shape.

## TAPERING

To cut a fine line into the head shape.

## TWIST CUTTING

Twist a 1 cm square section of hair and slide cut over the surface.

## UNDERCUTTING

The under panels of hair are shorter and do not technically check with the top sections.

## UNDERWRAP

To mix colour on the hair itself.

## V-SECTION CUTTING

To cut long narrow V-shapes into the lengths of each section of hair.

# Hairdressing And Beauty Industry Authority series – related titles

## Hairdressing

*Mahogany Hairdressing: Steps to Cutting, Colouring and Finishing Hair*
by Martin Gannon and Richard Thompson
*Mahogany Hairdressing: Advanced Looks*
*Essensuals, Next generation Toni & Guy: Step by Step*
*Patrick Cameron: Dressing Long Hair* by Patrick Cameron and Jacki Wadeson
*Patrick Cameron: Dressing Long Hair Book 2* by Patrick Cameron
*Bridal Hair* by Pat Dixon and Jacki Wadeson
*Trevor Sorbie: Visions in Hair* by Kris Sorbie and Jacki Wadeson
*The Total Look: The Style Guide for Hair and Make-Up Professionals* by Ian Mistlin
*Art of Hair Colouring* by David Adams and Jacki Wadeson

*Start Hairdressing: The Official Guide to Level 1* by Martin Green and Leo Palladino
*Hairdressing – The Foundations: The Official Guide to Level 2* by Leo Palladino
*Professional Hairdressing: The Official Guide to Level 3*
by Martin Green, Lesley Kimber and Leo Palladino
*Men's Hairdressing: Traditional and Modern Barbering* by Maurice Lister
*African-Caribbean Hairdressing* by Sandra Gittens
*The World of Hair: A Scientific Companion* by Dr John Gray
*Salon Management* by Martin Green

## Beauty Therapy

*Beauty Therapy – The Foundations: The Official Guide to Level 2*
by Lorraine Nordmann
*Professional Beauty Therapy: The Official Guide to Level 3*
by Lorraine Nordmann, Lorraine Appleyard and Pamela Linforth
*Aromatherapy for the Beauty Therapist* by Valerie Ann Worwood
*The World of Skin Care: A Scientific Companion* by Dr John Gray
*Indian Head Massage* by Muriel Burnham-Airey and Adele O'Keefe
*The Complete Nail Technician* by Marian Newman
*Safety in the Salon* by Elaine Almond